EXER-CISE WILL HURT YOU

EXER-CISE WILL HURT YOU

Concussion, Traumatic Brain Injury, and How the Dangers of Sports and Exercise Can Affect Your Health

STEVEN J. BARRER, MD

Seven Stories Press
New York • Oakland

A Seven Stories Press First Edition

Seven Stories Press
140 Watts Street
New York, NY 10013
www.sevenstories.com

College professors and high school and middle school teachers may order free examination copies of Seven Stories Press titles. To order, visit www.sevenstories.com/contact or send a fax on school letterhead to (212) 226-1411.

Library of Congress Cataloging-in-Publication Data
Barrer, Steven J.
  Exercise will hurt you : concussion, traumatic brain injury, and how the dangers of sports and exercise can affect your health / Steven J. Barrer, M.D.
     pages cm
  ISBN 978-1-60980-535-7 (hardback)
  1. Sports injuries. 2. Exercise--Health aspects. 3. Sports--Health aspects. 4. Medical misconceptions. I. Title.
  RD97.B36 2014
  617.1'027--dc23
                                        2014010249

Printed in the United States

9 8 7 6 5 4 3 2 1

For my children:

Hilary
Your courage inspires me,

Andrew
Dreams do come true,

Elisabeth
They cannot take you out of my mind or my heart.
I love you and miss you.

And for my wife Pam, who made all this possible,
and worth it.

CONTENTS

INTRODUCTION

I have never done anything athletic where I haven't hurt myself. Some of the injuries have been minor, others not so insignificant. Allow me to explain with a few examples.

Some years ago, while bicycling in a group, I broke my wrist—no minor injury for a surgeon. And I didn't even fall. My attention wandered for a moment and I rode onto the shoulder. The road surface was asphalt with a square-edged side that created a drop-off to the roadside that served as a culvert. It put me on a direct collision course with a drainage pipe that ran under a driveway just a few yards ahead of me. If I had collided with the pipe, my tire would have wedged into it, the bike would have come to an instantaneous halt, and I would have been catapulted over the handlebars.

In that surreal moment, just before disaster strikes and you know it's coming, time slows: I had a vivid picture of what was about to happen. The types of possible injuries flashed through my mind. It wasn't a question of whether or not there would be a crash. It was only a matter of how severe it would be.

In desperation, fueled by panic, I attempted to correct my course. With only a few microseconds to make a decision, I turned the bike back into the road edge, figuring it would cause me to fall. But sliding along the road surface still in contact with the bike would be preferable to being launched through the air.

It appeared at first to have succeeded. My front wheel struck the elevated road edge, causing the front tire to pop up in the air and land back on the road surface, and the rear tire followed. I was actually back on the road, still upright and even headed in the right direction. No one riding with me seemed to have even noticed.

The impact, however, caused a jarring that rippled up the bike's forward fork to the handlebars and fractured the scaphoid bone of my left wrist. At the time, I thought it was at worst a sprain. I didn't pay too much attention to the pain that at first was only mild. Mostly, I was overwhelmingly relieved that I would not require the local emergency medical services. I was also oddly proud of myself for having avoided what only seconds previously had loomed as a catastrophe. I finished the ride with my friends, loaded my bike back onto its carrier and drove home.

By that evening my wrist had become increasingly painful and swollen. I went to my hospital and had it x-rayed. I read the film myself and saw what looked like a fracture, but in my practice I rarely need to look at x-rays of the extremities. I had one of my emergency room colleagues look at it and he confirmed the break.

The scaphoid bone is one of eight that make up the wrist. It has a worrisome incidence of non-union, a situation where the bone does not heal, causing chronic pain, and in someone who works with his hands, disability.

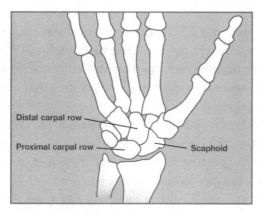

Scaphoid bone.

I consulted with my friend and hand surgeon, Bob Takei (yes, cousin of George Takei, Hikaru Sulu on 'Star Trek'), who gave me two options: I could wear a cast for twelve weeks, and if it didn't heal, undergo surgery to place a screw across the fracture, or go directly to the screw, in which case I'd be out of work for only four weeks.

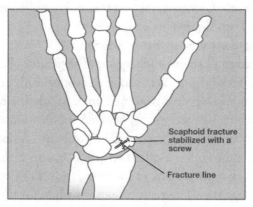

Illustration of screw in scaphoid bone.

The next day I had the surgery and was back in the operating room in two and a half weeks. Bob wasn't happy with my timeline but was pleased that it healed so well. Doctors make the worst patients, with the possible exception of nurses.

Why do I dwell on this injury? Because it, along with the rest of my personal history and more than thirty years of practicing medicine, has convinced me that, almost no matter what you do, exercise will hurt you.

Maybe I just have bad luck. My family tells me I'm injury-prone, though I suspect that's just a euphemism for people who do things that put them in harm's way. But a few years before the bike 'accident,' while playing third base for the hospital softball team, I reached down for a ground ball and heard a disturbing ripping sound from my calf. There was immediate pain and, shortly thereafter, discoloration above and behind my ankle indicating bleeding. I had torn my plantaris muscle, a small muscle that makes up part of the calf. I was on the disabled list for a month. Crutches, then a cane, and humiliation were my lot. I was injured playing *soft*ball.

Then there was my try at Aikido.

My cousin David Goldberg is a third-degree black belt of Aikido (and a master samurai swordsmith), and the sensei of his own dojo near my home. Aikido is a martial art in which you use your opponent's momentum against him: by redirecting your assailant's offensive action, you turn his move into an offensive action against himself. It is as much a philosophy of life as it is a form of combat. David suggested I come work out with him for the exercise. So I bought a ghee, looked very martial, and started down the path of health and self-defense. It didn't last a month. While doing a roll on the mats—there's lots of mat time in Aikido—I rolled onto my side with my arm tucked under me. The pressure of my ribs against the mat, with my elbow in between, cracked a rib—and another disturbing sound. Immediate pain, difficulty inhaling deeply, and another athletic endeavor terminated. Rib fractures hurt, a lot, and take months to heal completely. If you ever have one, try not to cough.

What else? There was the mild concussion playing neighborhood basketball, another torn calf muscle skiing in Colorado with a group of doctor friends from my hospital. Thank goodness for Paul Angotti, a podiatric surgeon who taped me up and at least got me ambulatory, if not exactly skiing. There was the day I played golf with my neighbor Bob Freedman. I was foolishly standing about twenty yards ahead of Bob, a very good golfer, but far enough to the side to feel safe. Not so. Bob hit the ball off the heel of the club, and it tracked directly at me like a heat-seeking missile. I tried to jump out of the way but was too close to have enough time to reach safety. The ball hit squarely on my shin. The pain was intense, as the thud that sounded like a cleaning wand whacking a carpet on a clothesline resounded in my ears. Bodily injuries make an amazingly diverse number of sounds. No broken bones this time, but a hematoma that went way beyond goose egg. The ball, of course, instead of ending up deep in the wooded rough where I was standing, careened back into the fairway, about a hundred yards ahead. After expressing his concern, Bob thanked me for the ricochet. Injured! While playing golf!

Then of course, there's my all-time favorite. While playing on my high school basketball team, I took a pass that bounced off my hands, striking dead on the two longest fingers that extended out from my open hands, the middle ones. Both broke at the last knuckle. They were chip fractures off the joint that required splinting in an extended position. Imagine the comments from my schoolmates as I walked the halls of high school with both middle fingers splinted in extension. I'd need to be writing a different kind of book to put most of them in print.

There have been other fractures: my collarbone twice, one toe, an index finger, and three ribs at two different times. Also there were any number of sprains, strains, pulls, contusions, abrasions, and lacerations that have accompanied my sports, exercise, and other physical activities over the years. While playing tennis, also in high school, I took a forehand slam to the eye, and still have the floaters that appeared after that.

So who am I? I'm a physician. More specifically, I am a neurosurgeon. I care for and operate on the brain, spine, and peripheral nerves. I have seen my share of athletic injuries to those body parts, and am expert in their care. I am not an orthopedic surgeon or a student of exercise physiology, physical medicine, rehabilitation, or muscle and joint injuries, which constitute, with the exception of the concussion, the entirety of my injuries. But I do see many head injuries every year. My hospital is a trauma center. Concussions, especially, have become hot news in recent years, claiming the careers of several prominent athletes. I've seen lots, as well as their more ominous cousins, cerebral contusions and hemorrhages, and skull fractures. I've seen the devastating and life-altering spinal cord injuries that occur primarily in contact sports, but also in diving accidents and, famously, horseback riding.

I've seen a career's worth of back pain, neck pain, arm and leg pain, altered gaits, and numb hands and feet that are the culmination of a lifetime's wear and tear on the human body. Many patients come to me when a sport or exercise can no longer be performed without causing pain, and they want the problem fixed. I remind them of the old joke about the patient who raises his arm and says "It hurts when I do this." "Don't do that," the doctor says. Patients are not amused. They want answers and cures.

The explanation is simple. We wear out. And the older we get, the more we wear. We just can't do at forty-five what came easily at twenty-five. And even those under twenty-five today often overdo it. Most patients, especially baby boomers like me, don't like the explanation. My generation is the first ever to incorporate exercise as a part of our lifestyles. My parents' generation, and those before them, did not. They didn't need to. They had more physical lifestyles. There were more laborers, more farmers; there was less access to mechanized transportation, and no electronic amusement for children. They went outside and played. And their food was healthier; fresher, less processed, frozen, packaged, and hormone- and antibiotic-infused. So as the boomers aged and became sedentary white-collar workers with questionable dietary habits, we took to the courts, fields, gyms, bikes, treadmills, and a hundred other pursuits in an effort to keep trim and fit. Many of us, and many of all ages, have taken this to extremes.

Researchers investigating the health effects of extreme exercise have studied participants in the Vasaloppet, a fifty-six-mile cross-country ski race that takes place yearly in Sweden. Among the questions asked is how the long-term health of these athletes was affected.[1] In the June 2013 issue of the *European Heart Journal,* Dr. Kasper Andersen, a cardiologist at Uppsala University Hospital (Uppsala, Sweden), and lead author of a study looking at the cardiac health of more than fifty-two thousand Vasaloppet participants, said: "We found that those who completed five or more races in a period of ten years, had a 30% higher risk of developing any arrhythmia (a problem with the rhythm or rate of the heartbeat) than those who did one race only. Similarly, skiers who had the fastest finishing time relative to the other participants also had a 30% higher risk of developing any arrhythmia in subsequent years."[2]

Picking up on the staggering implications of the Andersen study, Gretchen Reynolds writing for the *New York Times* online in July 2013, asked, "Can you get too much exercise?"[3] It seems intuitive that something that is good for you is even better if you can get more of it. Not always so. In my profession certainly, medication is prescribed in very specific dosages that are carefully worked out for efficacy and safety. In the same way that a medication that is good for you at a certain dose can be quite dangerous at a higher dose, too much exercise can have a ruinous, even life-threatening effect on a person's health.

Why the heart problems were found in extreme exercisers is unclear. One possible explanation may be the anatomic changes seen in the hearts of older aggressive exercisers. In a 2011 study published in the Journal of Applied Physiology, investigators found an unexpectedly high prevalence of myocardial fibrosis (scarring of the heart) in lifelong, competitive endurance athletes over fifty years of age.[4] Scarring of the myocardium, or heart wall, is associated with cardiac arrhythmias.

Support for this theory comes from the University of Montreal. Published in the *Journal of the American College of Cardiology* in July 2013, Gausch and associates studied the hearts of rats subjected to exercise training. They found that the animals' hearts developed atrial dilatation (enlargement of the upper heart chambers), and, as in the human study, fibrosis. These rats had increased susceptibility to atrial fibrillation, a heart arrhythmia, linking the findings of exercise-associated changes in cardiac anatomy and exercise-associated arrhythmias.[5] Atrial fibrillation in humans is a treatable disease. Although it can have serious consequences, most notably stroke, long-term control is the rule.

What all this means to the long-term overall health of those who exercise vigorously is unclear. In general, any increased susceptibility to cardiac disease is associated with a shorter life expectancy. However, Reynolds in her *Times* article quotes another animal study in exercised rats that showed a lower incidence of ventricular fibrillation, a highly lethal form of cardiac arrhythmia. Published in June 2013, in *PLOS ONE*, thirty rats were divided into three groups: sedentary, short- term trained, and long-term trained animals. The ability to induce ventricular fibrillation was diminished in the exercise-trained rats, with the lowest incidence in the long-term trained hearts.[6]

What the relationship is between the animal results and the findings in humans from the Vasaloppet study is speculative. And the results of the two exercised rat studies are somewhat contradictory. As Reynolds points out, quoting one of the authors of the Montreal study, it's possible that the animals in the ventricular fibrillation study that were exercised at a lower intensity and for fewer weeks than the rats in the Montreal study hadn't yet developed the fibrosis seen in the Montreal rats, and therefore evidenced only exercise benefits.

Exercise training for the heart has a long and well-studied history of providing a benefit to the health and well-being of the active individual. There is an enormous literature supporting this well-established fact. But as the above studies show, and as I will illustrate in this book, there is another side to the story. I posit that exercise can be bad for you in several ways. Injuries can result from routine participation in sport and exercise, even at the most basic level. And there are hidden dangers that lie in the cumulative effect of even the seemingly most trivial of injuries or just the overuse of our joints and muscles in the absence of injury. So, can you get too much exercise?

Later in these pages, I will present the stories of two celebrated runners who died from cardiac disease at relatively young ages. Certainly there are any number of counter-stories of individuals who have benefited from being vigorous exercisers; every reader of this book probably knows several such people. This research provides a glimpse into the possible reasons why, sometimes, exercise is bad for you.

I wrote this book for two reasons. I hate to exercise.

This fact will be apparent throughout the stories that involve me. I am also physically lazy, and this too will be clear to you. I no longer make apologies for these personality traits. I used to be embarrassed by them and envied my friends who were more disciplined with exercise, but it's not for lack of trying. I've described some of my athletic exploits above, and my foray into organized exercise workouts will follow. I simply have never been able to stay with them. I could not overcome my inherent dislike of exercise, and I especially disliked the pain of the injuries.

Over time, I also came to the realization that I am not an exception. Many people think like I do. Even among my colleagues, doctors who are supposed to know better and dispense advice about the importance of staying active, there was an attitude held by some that exercise is a necessary evil, emphasis on the word "evil." I found the same thing with many people I spoke to about this issue. It was a revelation. Suddenly there were lots of people just like me. It's empowering. I wasn't alone in my embarrassment; there were others I could confess to and find support rather than derision. We didn't know about each other because no one, especially among doctors, wants to talk about it. So I decided to embrace my feelings about exercise and stop apologizing for them. It is simply who I am, and it is unlikely I will ever be able to change. I've contemplated starting a support group for the exercise-challenged. I could apply for 501(c)(3) status under the Internal Revenue Code. It covers charitable groups including religious, educational, amateur athletic, scientific, literary, and public safety organizations, as well as those involved in the prevention of cruelty to children and animals. I figure I could justify qualification on the basis of several of those categories including educational (self-explanatory), amateur athletic (or its antithesis), public safety (avoid injury!), and especially the prevention of cruelty (to me).

Or, I could write a book.

Which brings me to the other reason I wrote this book: to bring some reason to the cult of exercise, which is indeed fraught with potential dangers, some obvious and some less so, as seen in the above-mentioned Vasaloppet and Gausch studies of the effect of extreme exercise on the heart. As a surgeon, I am ethically and legally bound to provide my patients with informed consent prior to proceeding with an operation. I recommend surgery every day; it is, after all, what I do for a living. I determine that I can fix a patient's problem surgically and explain in detail why I think that is so, pointing out what the problem is, and how the operation will correct it. I routinely use pictures and illustrations, often from my textbooks or charts specifically designed to explain a given problem. The patient's imaging studies, scans and x-rays, show the patient what he or she has, and aid in understanding what I am recommending. I provide percentages for the odds of success of surgery and explain that sometimes the surgery fails, and why that may be.

Fully informed consent requires of me that I explain, in excruciating detail, what can go wrong with surgery. If the patient is unable to understand what I'm saying, I must also explain it to the legal guardian. If the patient does not speak English, I am legally bound to give the explanation through a certified medical translator fluent in both languages. If he or she is deaf, I have to have a signer present. The discussion must include all the common risks that are intuitive with surgery, such as infection, wound-healing problems, and bleeding. But there are the less common risks like anesthesia complications and medication and blood transfusion reactions. In my specialty, where surgery is on the brain and spine, potential complications are particularly frightful. Operating on the brain can leave one paralyzed, blind, or unable to speak, swallow, or hear. Surgery on the spine can render a patient wheelchair-bound and forever dependent on others. Although those are all rare complications, with elective neurosurgery of all types having extremely low complication rates, there is usually a pause on the part of the patient before signing the consent form. In my practice, I have all this information printed on forms that patients are given to keep. I never want a patient to feel that I haven't explained everything they need to know in deciding on a treatment course, especially a surgical one. The forms also state that I gave the patient the opportunity to ask questions, and that I answered them to the patient's satisfaction.

In all the years I have been buying exercise equipment, weight machines, ridiculously expensive road bikes, tread mills, running shoes and all the rest, no salesman, not a single one, ever told me how the activity for which I was making the purchase might harm me. There is no 'informed consent' doctrine in exercise and sports equipment retail sales.

There should be. "Let the buyer beware" may be a time-honored maxim of commerce, but it doesn't apply to ladders, cigarettes, drugs, children's wading pools, plastic bags, diving boards, car air bags, alcohol, or extension cords and toys with small pieces that could fit in a child's mouth, among others. And of course, it doesn't apply to surgery. It shouldn't apply to exercise either.

Look at a ladder sometime. There are warning labels pasted to virtually every inch of the ladder's surface. If you read them, you'd never even get on the first step. Unfortunately, I didn't look at them until afterwards. On the weekend before hurricane Sandy slammed the Northeast in October 2012, I was on a ladder cleaning out my gutters. Sandy was technically classified as a tropical cyclone with winds as high as 115 mph. Cyclone sounds scarier than hurricane (although meteorologically they're the same weather phenomenon). I had the ladder leaning against the edge of the roof with my hands in the decaying muck of dead leaves that had been lying in the gutters since the previous winter. The ladder began to slip, slowly at first, but gathered speed. It was a long ladder, extending about five feet above the roof. Since it was sliding without tilting, I decided to ride it down until I was closer to the ground before jumping off, and before the ladder cleared the edge and fell to the ground. My leap was controlled and from only two or three feet, but I landed on my feet in such a way that I fractured my right ankle.

The pain was like being stabbed and caused me to fall backwards on my asphalt driveway. Fearing that I'd hit my head on the hard surface, (that's the first thing a neurosurgeon thinks about in such a situation), I tucked my chin to keep the back of my head elevated. Safe, I thought, and popped up glad to not be concussed, only to collapse again from the pain in my foot.

Although this injury didn't come from exercising, it does serve as an example of what one can face when not fully informed. When the pain subsided enough to allow me to walk, I went to the shed to read the ladder. The warnings are largely common sense and logical. There is one that states "failure to read and follow instructions on this ladder may result in injuries or death." It is accompanied by a little picture of a man falling off a ladder, arms and legs flailing. In my defense, it doesn't specifically mention ankle fractures.

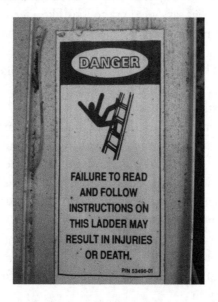

This book provides for the exerciser a basis for informed consent. It is, in the phrase journalist Paul Harvey famously coined, "the rest of the story." I will discuss some of the more common hazards in detail and point out ways to avoid them. After all, there are benefits to exercise, and even the most skeptical part of me realizes that exercise will always be with us. But thousands of other authors have written that story. That exercise is good for you is as ingrained in the American psyche as the wholesomeness of apple pie. I hope to convince you that there is room for moderation and common sense in exercise, because it can and will harm you. There are far more injuries that arise from exercise and sport each year than from surgery.[7] Most of all, I hope to help you realize that you need to pay attention to your body and not to the marketing that says you have to look like a teenager when you are at retirement age. Having an abdominal six pack at sixty just isn't worth it if you have to beat yourself up to get it. The same goes for fifty and forty. I like to think the sixth sense is common sense. This book is an appeal to your sixth sense.

A final introductory thought: I use humor in this book both to make it enjoyable to read and to counterbalance the serious side. I've learned there has to be a barrier between the physician and the often serious, sometimes life-threatening conditions we treat in order for sanity to prevail. There are many ways to create that separation, and humor is a way I deal with it. So please forgive me for any of the places in this book where I may seem inappropriately light-hearted. It is how I've survived for the past forty-one years.

Chapter 1

THE CULT OF EXERCISE AND THE MECHANICS OF INJURY

In the introduction I described how the Baby Boomer generation has made exercise a part of their lifestyle. Why? Where did this come from? People have always exercised and played sports. Yoga is an ancient art. The Olympics are thousands of years old. Every ancient culture that has been excavated has shown evidence of sport competition. The indigenous tribal populations of North America played a form of lacrosse that showed up in their legends and was documented as early as the seventeenth century.[1] Maimonides, a thirteenth century Jewish scholar and physician, wrote about both diet and exercise. He recommended exercise before eating to encourage the building of muscle rather than fat and also had specific ideas about how to eat for good health.[2]

And then there is the 1975 movie *The Man Who Would be King*. On their way to conquer the fictional country of Kafiristan, two soldiers of fortune (played by Michael

Caine and Sean Connery) defeat a warlord whose people play a form of polo that uses the head of a defeated enemy wrapped in a bag as the object to get between the goal posts. When there are no sporting goods stores one must improvise. I can imagine that severed-head polo may not be far from the reality of some of the games played by the less genteel societies of yesteryear.

While on vacation in Costa Rica some years ago, our guide told me all that was needed to start a village in that country was a church, a bar, and a soccer field. At least two of the three are positive institutions. I'll let you choose which two.

Such is the influence that sport and physical activity have had on the development of the world's civilizations. Movie-making too. Everyone participates in some sort of sporting activity at some point in his or her life. Even the physically challenged have developed ways to join in; for example, through the Paralympic Games. In recent decades the Special Olympics, for children and adults with developmental challenges, has evolved into a world-wide organization of great merit. Eunice Kennedy Shriver has spearheaded much of that evolution.

It's not entirely clear where the origins of the modern exercise phenomenon lie. It is certainly a product of the twentieth century, likely its first half. And there is no single individual who can claim the title of father of the movement, but there are a few candidates. The history is fascinating if somewhat murky. The personalities are large and well-known to those of us who grew up reading their claims of how their exercise programs could turn us from ninety-eight-pound weaklings into muscle-bound Adonises who would never lack for beautiful women hanging onto our sculpted biceps. The roots may actually spring from the world of nutrition, as we'll see from what follows.

Paul Bragg, according to his personal story, was born in 1881 and raised on a homestead in Virginia. According to legend, he looked hale and hearty to the end of his life, younger than his ninety-five years. He died in 1976. Bragg is credited with bringing the dangers of an unhealthy diet to the attention of the public and became famous, and rich, by touting the benefits of health food. He told his personal story and extolled the wisdom of his nutritional theories in several books and countless interviews.

At age sixteen, he contracted tuberculosis, generally considered to be a fatal disease in 1897. He was cured by Dr. August Rollier in his TB clinic in Switzerland, using holistic treatments including exercise, outdoor sunshine, and fasting.[3] The positive health effects of those simple measures were a revelation to Bragg, and he brought that experience back to the United States and developed it into a worldwide phenomenon that persists to this day.

He went on to become a world-class athlete and competed in two Olympic games in 1908 and 1912 on the US wrestling team, fought in the trenches of World War I, played tennis with Teddy Roosevelt, and taught the President's sons to box. He began his nutritional empire by opening the first health food store in America in 1912. His dietary theories revolved around fasting and using water and juices to maintain hydration. Natural supplements that he called "live food" replaced the usual American diet, much of which, according to Bragg, came out of a frying pan.

One can still find his products for sale. Organic apple cider vinegar, organic extra virgin olive oil, salad dressings, and seasonings constitute the more popular products. His Liquid Aminos—mostly a soy solution with a variety of amino acids added—is touted as a great addition to virtually any food you can think of.

Bragg was one of the first to raise the specter of fluoridated water being an insidious, government-sponsored health hazard. Due to his self-promoted high profile, he became a nutritional consultant to the rich and famous, especially those in Hollywood. The year before he died he was asked in a *People* magazine interview when sexual activity ended. "You'll have to ask someone else. I'm only ninety-four," he answered. He is also credited with having been the inspiration for Jack LaLanne, arguably the first of the famous exercise gurus. More about him later.

Sadly, it's likely that almost none of Bragg's personal story is true. In his 2007 article, "Paul Bragg's Tarnished Legacy," writer Wade Frazier, himself a former follower of the nutritional advice of Bragg, lays out the evidence for the fraudulent nature of the nutritionist's claims. The author starts with pictures of Bragg, including one taken in 1932 when he would have been fifty-one. "He looked like a Greek god, a deeply tanned, muscle-bound man in his thirties . . ." Since Photoshop was still a half-century away, either his nutritional regimen really was miraculous, or he had lied about his age, and was in fact in his thirties. We all know someone who lies about his or her age to make us think they're younger than reality. I always thought it made more sense to reverse that. If I tell someone I'm seventy-eight when in fact I'm sixty-four, the response I get is "Wow, you look great!" It seems Bragg came up with that idea long before I did. Frazier adds that in his last years, photos of Bragg in his books appeared to have been airbrushed.

A variety of other documents, including census and immigration records, Bragg's draft card, and a variety of newspaper articles also pointed Frazier in the direction of a fabricated history. The U.S. census of 1900 lists a Paul C. Bragg as having been born in 1895 in Indiana; not in Virginia in 1881. It has been suggested by some that there could be two Paul C. Braggs in the world, but Bragg's draft card, unequivocally his and signed by him, confirms the 1895 date and Indiana location of his birth. It additionally lists his profession as a life insurance salesman. His birth certificate and the newspaper announcement of his birth also give the date and location of his birth as 1895 in Indiana.

On his draft card, he requested an exemption from serving in Europe during WWI, citing his service in the National Guard for the previous three years and the fact that he had a dependent wife. His having served in any battles in the trenches therefore is likely untrue.

Given the evidence of his later-than-claimed birth date, Bragg would have been only thirteen at the time of the 1908 Olympics, and seventeen for the 1912 games. Although there has been the rare Olympian of such young ages, based on available records, Bragg's name was not on the roster of the US wrestling team in either Olympiad. Another significant discrepancy in the dating of Bragg's personal history is the cure of his TB. Based on his claim of birth in 1881 and his stated age when treated at the

Swiss clinic, he would have left there in 1898. August Rollier did not found his clinic until 1903.

Given the above evidence, as well as additional information in Frazier's essay, creating an alternative reality appeared to come easily to Paul Bragg. Insurance salesmen of that era were considered disreputable, and the industry little more than a scam. Some would say, and I count myself among them, that the nutritional supplement industry is, in many respects, also a scam, particularly in relation to diet and weight loss supplements. Going from insurance to nutrition then may not have been that much of a leap for Bragg, and as a result, all his claims regarding his nutritional theories are tarnished by the duplicity of his autobiographical history. His age above all appears to have been fabricated, so although he looked great when he died at his claimed age of ninety-five, he only looked so-so for an eighty-one year old.

There may be some truth to some of Bragg's claims about his health foods. Unfortunately, both for him and all the others that followed, efficacy is difficult to determine. Nutritional supplements that are natural products, those that come from plants, herbs, and animal products that exist in nature, what Bragg called live food, are not subjected to scrutiny by the Food and Drug Administration (FDA). Synthetically manufactured products designed to be ingested by or implanted into the human body, such as medications, medical treatments, and surgically implanted devices, are required to undergo rigorous, time-consuming and expensive trials that must prove efficacy and safety. The trials are closely monitored by experts in the appropriate fields and must conform to accepted standards of scientific research. It usually takes several years to complete the process, and if the FDA feels the product has not met the necessary standards, it cannot be brought to market, and the investment is lost.

There is no such requirement for naturally occurring substances. As such, the claims as to what they can provide to the user are often exaggerated and not supported by the same type of research required by the FDA of synthetic substances. The consumer remains insufficiently informed.

It may seem that I have gone somewhat far afield from the subject of exercise. But this background is key to understanding the origins of the exercise industry. Exercise and nutrition go hand-in-hand. An important part of Bragg's thesis for good health was the inclusion of regular exercise. And Bragg is considered to have strongly influenced one of the earliest pioneers of what has become a multi-billion dollar industry.

Jack LaLanne was that pioneer. His website refers to him as the "Godfather of Fitness." His biography reveals an early life similar to Bragg's claimed childhood. LaLanne's, however, is true. He was born to poor French immigrant parents in Oakland in 1914. His *New York Times* obituary describes him as an "emotional and physical wreck while growing up in the San Francisco area." When he was fifteen he heard Bragg lecture on the benefits of exercise and a healthy diet, and it transformed his life.

He built an empire that eclipsed Bragg's. He began to exercise with free weights, and in 1936 opened a fitness spa in Oakland that incorporated a fitness gym with a juice bar and health food store, the prototype for the thousands that followed.[4] By 1951 he was on local television with a fitness show that later went nationwide in 1959. The show continued until the mid-1980s. Along the way he sold his proprietary electric juicer and exercise devices, brought women into the exercise culture, produced books and exercise videos, and convinced the elderly that they too could benefit from exercise and stay the ravages of old age.

He became a national celebrity. At age sixty and again at seventy, he performed swimming feats where he towed boats while covering more than a mile in the water. He expanded his empire by opening fitness studios around the country, ultimately licensing them to Bally.[5]

Dear to my heart is the fact that LaLanne was known to say that he didn't like to exercise. The effect on his health and well-being, however, drove him on.

Another name that is closely associated both with fitness and this time period is Charles Atlas. He too has been given the title of founding father of the exercise industry, and in his peak years was described as having the world's most perfect body. His origins follow the now familiar refrain. Born Angelo Siciliano in Italy in 1893, he emigrated with his parents at age ten. In his books and interviews he described himself in his teenage years as being feeble and sickly, a ninety-eight-pound weakling. I always thought the iconic vignette of the skinny kid sitting on the beach with his girlfriend, getting sand kicked in his face by the muscled bully, was the stuff of comic book stories. Apparently that is exactly what happened to Angelo on a beach in Coney Island, except that he weighed ninety-seven pounds.[6]

Humiliated, he took his initial inspiration to achieve

the perfect body from the statues of the Greek gods he saw while visiting the Brooklyn Museum. Working with crude weights and elastic bands, he tried to build himself into what he saw in the statues, but with no success. His next revelation came from the Bronx Zoo, where he studied a male lion as it went through its stretching routine. In Charles Gaines and George Butler's biography of him—*Yours in a Perfect Manhood*—Atlas describes that moment as the seed for an exercise philosophy that turned his body into one envied worldwide and that launched his own fitness empire.

He realized that the lion's stretching was a form of exercise, working one muscle against another—what in time would become known as isometric exercise. He took this lesson home and on his own invented a full exercise routine that was born of his observation of the lion. This time it worked. He developed an enviable physique that led a friend to describe him as looking like the statue of Atlas atop the Atlas Hotel, coining the name he would take as his own, adding an American first name to become Charles Atlas.[7]

Unlike his contemporaries, Atlas had no thoughts at that time of turning his personal success into a career. He might have receded into obscurity had he not been noticed by an artist on a beach in 1916, and asked to pose. Then he was introduced to socialite Gertrude Vanderbilt Whitney, a sculptor and patron of the arts, and never looked back. He was soon in demand and posed for some of the most famous statuary in the country, gracing venues such as Washington Square Park, Queens Borough Hall, the Elk's national headquarters, and Washington, DC.

Photos of him appeared everywhere, "in classic poses, nude or shockingly close to it and with more than a whiff of eroticism, suggest[ing] how much he liked the camera and the camera liked him."[8]

He parlayed his photogenic fame into wins in two photo contests, "World's Most Beautiful Man," and "World's Most Perfectly Developed Man." His looks and toned body however, did not translate into business acumen. With a contact he met at this time he started a mail-order business to sell exercise equipment that nearly failed. In 1928, he met Charles Roman, who had been assigned Atlas' account at the advertising agency that represented his company. Within months, Roman had revived the business and Atlas, impressed and smart enough to recognize an opportunity, offered him half the company on the condition that he would run it.[9]

The rest is the stuff of legend. Like Bragg and LaLanne, Atlas, with Roman, built the business into an enormous success.

And therein lies the basic fuel of the exercise industry. It has made lots of people lots of money. The men highlighted above are just a few of the many who have had, and still have, lucrative careers from selling and promoting nutrition and exercise. I am not implying that all those who promote health are insincere and have only profit as motive, only some of them.

Bragg is an example of the latter. He has been proven to have promoted himself fraudulently. And I have outlined how the nutritional supplement and diet industry can circumvent accepted science while promoting their products with, in some cases, promises of results that rival those offered by the snake oil salesmen of the Old West.

LaLanne and Atlas, on the other hand, were sincere. They appear to have strongly believed in their message, served as living examples, and felt they were helping the millions who signed on to their programs. Those who knew him described Atlas as a humble man. Despite great wealth, ostentatiously displayed by his partner Roman, Atlas lived a simple life. Throughout his life, home was a four-room fifth-floor Brooklyn apartment he shared with his wife and two children. He was philanthropic and a strong promoter of the Boy Scouts. Although he "seemed to love the limelight," was often seen in the company of the beautiful and famous, and was a constant self-promoter, there is no indication that he was in any way mendacious or had any less than full faith in the positive effects of his methods.[10]

That being said, here is a number to ponder: 180,000,000,000. Since I never said there'd be math in this book, that number is 180 billion, with a 'b.' And, that number is in dollars. Estimates vary, but with some minor variation that number is the sum of $40 billion spent on dietary products, $75 billion for nutritional supplements, $15 billion spent on exercise equipment, and $50 billion on gym memberships in this country every year.[11] Each year! And that doesn't include the accessories: clothing, food processing devices, spa vacations, travel, and medical care for the mishaps. I should know. I've contributed my share to that sum. Of the 15 percent of Americans who have gym memberships, only 8 percent actually use them.[12] I should know. I have one I don't use.

There's nothing wrong with success. This is, after all, America. Rags to riches, Horatio Alger, the American dream; it's the iconic story of the many thousands of people who have risen from poverty. Bragg, LaLanne, and Atlas are examples. They had an idea, some might say a revelation, developed it passionately, promoted it relentlessly, and reaped the financial benefits. Ayn Rand would have been proud and probably was. She was a contemporary.

They have served as prominent examples to those who have followed them. And there are many. Exercise franchises, videos, television exercise workouts, reality shows and promotional advertising, health food and nutritional stores, and social media all have fueled the industry's growth. The Internet even gave new life to the products and promotions of the three pioneers who had faded and been eclipsed by the 1970s and 1980s. Sales are booming again despite all three being gone.

In all endeavors, if there are fortunes to be made, they will be. This is especially true if the endeavor in question is perceived as being good for participants. The fitness industry is one such example and as a result floats many boats. Equipment manufacturing, service, fashion, food, vitamins, and supplements are a few of the feeder industries whose health has improved as we have improved ours. Holistic living styles and medical therapies are becoming more popular. When I discuss treatment options with my patients who have problems that don't require one specific course of treatment, I routinely include alternative medicine. Acupuncture is the most common one, primarily for patients with various types of pain. I have no idea how it works, but for some it does. As long as the needles are sterile and the patient doesn't have a bleeding disorder, at least it will do no harm.

There has been a reemergence of ancient Eastern forms of medicine that have been practiced for thousands of years, in part as a result of the popularity of nutrition and fitness. Natural healing is gaining traction within holistic medicine, and there are now naturopathic medical schools in nine states and two Canadian provinces. Their curricula are heavily weighted with natural healing methods and the prescription of what Bragg called live foods. Their graduates are licensed to establish general medical practices, and some medical insurance companies will cover their services.

Mainstream medicine has not been left out. Within recent decades, the medical subspecialty of sports medicine has come into being. Prominent in this arena are orthopedic surgeons, but physiatry (physical medicine and rehabilitation) and family medicine offer fellowship training in this discipline as well. It involves the evaluation and treatment of a broad variety of injury types, but deals primarily with injuries of the joints, especially to the soft tissues associated with them—ligaments, tendons, and cartilaginous structures. Physical therapy is the mainstay of this medical care using rest, bracing, and anti-inflammatory medication early in the process. Modalities such as ice or heat, aqua-therapy, electrical stimulation, ultrasound, and massage, among others, are at times helpful. Once pain permits, active and passive stretching—exercise to return tone and strength and gradual rehabilitation—take the athlete back to the point where he or she can return to play.

Fractures fall under the care of general orthopedic surgeons and when a joint has been worn out beyond the ability of non-surgical care to help, the joint replacement orthopedic surgeons step in.

Spine and head injuries are cared for by neurosurgeons like me, although some orthopedists care for the injured spine too. And there has been an explosion of information on mild traumatic brain injury, the most common being concussions, to the point that my hospital, under my direction, established a concussion referral service for the area schools to deal with the increasing number of concussed student athletes. Unfortunately, business is booming. More about that in a later chapter.

To paraphrase Garret Morris' comic take on Latin American baseball players during his stint on 'Saturday Night Live,' "exercise been veddy veddy good to America." The exercise craze has been good for the economy, creating an industry that didn't exist until less than a hundred years ago. I've alluded to the many spin-offs, from fashion to head injury; quite a broad spectrum. For better or worse, the impact of exercise has been enormous on this country.

Let's look at some of the consequences of that impact.

SPRAINS, STRAINS, PULLS AND TEARS

I could fill this book with the soft tissue injuries that accompany every sport and exercise imaginable. With absolutely no reliable data to support it, my educated guess would put the incidence of these kinds of injuries at 100 percent; more than that actually, if one assumes, as I do, that most of us have had more than one. I described two muscle injuries that I've had, and there have been lots more. Sprained ankles and jammed fingers seemed to be part of my friends' and my childhood playing peewee football, Little League baseball, and backyard everything. The sore backs, painful joints and aching muscles that have accompanied my later-in-life weekend warrior days are legion.

It turns out there indeed may be reliable data. Yang and associates, at the University of Iowa, looked at the epidemiology of overuse and acute injuries in collegiate athletes.[13] They used the definitions of Albright and others.[14] Overuse injuries are those of gradual onset caused by repetitive trauma. There is no single, definable event causative of a specific injury. An acute injury is defined as one caused by a specific, recognizable event. To be included in the study, the injury had to have clinical signs of tissue damage and the injured player had to have been unable to return to play on the same day.

Included among overuse injuries are bursitis, deformity, impingement, inflammation, joint laxity, stress fractures and tendinitis. Examples of acute injuries are vascular injuries, fractures, dislocations, nerve injuries, open wounds, sprains and strains. There are others of both types.

In the three years over which the study was conducted, the results found 573 athletes who sustained 1,317 injuries. Almost a third of the injuries were of the overuse type; 386 or 30 percent, of which the most common were general stress, inflammation and tendonitis, in that order. The majority, 931 or 70 percent, were acute injuries, most commonly sprains and strains.[15]

In their discussion of the study results, the authors list several limitations. The first was the possibility that the athletes who have overuse injuries, those in which there is no discernible single injury, under-report their symptoms. They may be self treating, underestimating the seriousness of their injury, or unwilling to notify trainers and coaches for fear of losing playing time. The actual number of this type of injure could therefore be higher than found by the authors.

Supporting this supposition is the work of Clarsen and colleagues from the Trauma Research Center of the Norwegian School of Sport Sciences. They developed a new, more robust method for monitoring the number of overuse injuries in athletes.[16] They start with the observations that these injuries receive scant attention in the literature of sports related injuries, reliable data on their number and seriousness are scarce, and few studies deal with their prevention. They provide as an explanation the nature of these injuries: pains often assumed to be a natural part of training and playing, the often minimal discomfort early in the injury's development, and the ability to continue to play in the early phase of the problem. Athletes may not report as an injury a condition they feel to be a normal part of participating in their sport.

These authors note that most studies of overuse injuries monitor only injuries that result in time lost from practice or play. A better method, they propose, would be to monitor a continuum of injury. Quoting a 2009 study from the *British Journal of Sports Medicine* that stated that injuries that don't cause lost time from competition are rarely used in injury studies, Clarsen et al. proposed to register three categories of injury: 'any physical complaint,' 'medical attention,' and 'time-loss.'[17] They developed a registry that included this broader spectrum of injury definition and used it to collect injury data that was then compared to the same athlete's injuries registered in more traditional databases.

A total of 313 elite Norwegian athletes completed the questionnaires developed for this study. There were a variety of sports; cross-country skiing, floorball, handball, road cycling and volleyball. Using the standard method of data acquisition, a total of 103 time-loss injuries were recorded among 82 athletes, 42 acute injuries and 61 overuse injuries. The data collection using the new method of registration found 236 athletes (75 percent of the cohort) who reported an injury. A total of 419 overuse injuries were reported in these 236 study subjects. For reasons that are not addressed in the study, acute injuries were not part of the new method of data collection. It would be logical, therefore, to assume that more than 75 percent of the cohort sustained injury.

The authors use the 'tip of the iceberg' analogy to introduce their theory that current methodologies of injury research significantly underestimate the magnitude of the problem. Their results suggest validation of that theory. Future investigations will need to take these study results into account.

Almost everyone knows about sprains, strains, pulls and tears. If you haven't had one, you are a rare individual indeed. Most are similar regardless of the activity that causes them. But these are real injuries, with a specific pathophysiology, and are not always minor. A tear of the anterior cruciate ligament (ACL) of the knee, to name arguably the best-known example, is often a career-ending event. Let's talk about these kinds of injuries here in detail, as a class of injury encountered in all forms of sport and exercise.

Tendons and ligaments are bands of fibrous connective tissue that serve to hold us together. Tendons are found at each end of a skeletal muscle and attach it to bone. Ligaments attach bones to each other where they meet to form joints. In some joints such as the knee, where there is no inherent stability of the joint, the ligaments and tendons provide all of it.

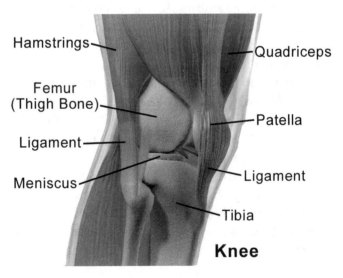

Anatomy of the knee.

Other joints—for example, the hip or shoulder that are ball-in-socket joints—are less inherently unstable but no less susceptible to injuries of their connective tissue.

Tendon tears, also called ruptures, are commonly known as strains. Ligament tears are known as sprains. Both of these are incomplete tears. A complete tear is more serious and separation of either of these structures from its attachment to bone is called an avulsion. There are three degrees of injury based on severity. First degree is the least severe; third degree is the most severe and includes full thickness tears and avulsions.

These tears in the tendons and ligaments initiate the inflammatory process, a complicated cellular cascade that the body uses to repair damaged tissue. The injury causes immediate anatomic damage to the connective tissue substrate of the tendon/ligament. There is both vascular disruption causing bleeding and nerve injury causing immediate and, at times, excruciating pain. It's difficult to forget the image of an injured athlete writhing on the ground holding his knee or ankle, his face contorted by the agony of this kind of injury. Within hours of the injury, a fluid collects around the torn fibers that contains many of the cellular elements that establish inflammation.

There are five clinical hallmarks of inflammation that every medical student learns in the first year of medical school. They are, in Latin: *rubor* (redness), *calor* (heat), *dolor* (pain), *tumor* (swelling) and *functio laesa* (loss of function). The first four were recognized and described by Celsus in the first century C.E., and Galen added the fifth element in the second century. Both lived and wrote in Rome. Little is known about Celsus and few of his writings survive, although his name is attached to a scale of temperature measurement. Galen was a well-known physician in his time and many of his writings, much of them incorrect, guided medical education until the six-teenth century.

Treatment of sprains and strains is directed at both the injury and the inflammation that results. The initial treatments are all anti-inflammatory. Ice reduces swelling, lowers temperature and is an analgesic, thereby addressing three of the five components. Elevation further reduces swelling, which has the secondary effect of reducing pain; tissue that is tense and expanded from swelling is a pain generator of its own. Anti-inflammatory medications slow the cellular response that creates inflammation, and they have a direct analgesic effect beyond that which comes with the slowed inflammation.

It may seem counterproductive to treat the inflamma-tion of an injury with drugs that slow the very process that produces the healing of the injured tissue. There is a degree of cognitive dissonance among physicians as a result. The assumption is that the inflammatory process has run amok, and goes into overdrive after an injury. The use of anti-inflammatory medications reduces the inten-sity of the response enough to ease the pain, but not so far as to stop the healing process all together. There is recent research, however, that suggests these medications do indeed interfere with healing. Two studies found that ibuprofen, the ingredient in many of the commonly used NSAIDs (non-steroidal anti-inflammatory drugs) includ-ing Motrin and Advil, slowed recovery in an injured rat tendon, inhibiting both the proliferation of tendon cells[18] and protein synthesis.[19] A third study confirmed the slowed healing seen in injuries treated with all NSAIDs tested except ibuprofen and acetaminophen, the active ingredient in Tylenol, which is not an anti-inflammatory but an analgesic only.[20]

The studies used an animal model, and it's always uncertain whether one can make the leap from rats to humans in applying scientific research results. Although it seems intuitive that the studies are accurate, and I'm not sure that it makes sense why ibuprofen gets a pass, I'm glad it does because I use it by the wheelbarrow full. I recommend it as a first line drug in virtually every patient I see with a pain problem. In my experience, it is as effective as any of the other medications in this drug class, and it's the least expensive, especially when ordered as the generic form. Many of my colleagues feel the same way. We call it 'vitamin M,' for its trade name Motrin. It can be obtained over-the-counter without prescription, and, although convenient, in proprietary form it is the most expensive way to buy it. I keep a three-hundred-count jar of the generic USP form of it in my medicine cabinet at all times, and I never leave home without it. I use it most commonly for headache but the recommended dose of four hundred milligrams is insufficient for anyone weighing more than a hundred pounds. Six or eight hundred mg. is what I take for pain. But don't take my word on this. Ask your physician and then make your own informed decision.

Rest and immobilization are essential to allow healing to occur. Within days, actual tissue healing begins. Granulation tissue starts to form at the injury site. Most of us have seen this in a cut or wound that remains open and heals from the bottom up. It is red-pink in color and has a bumpy appearance, hence its name. Granulation tissue contains macrophages, fibroblasts, and vascular growth factor, the cellular factors that regenerate the damaged tissue. By about the fifth day, new collagen, the basic substrate of tendons and ligaments, has started to form. The early phase of this process is disorganized, but as the forming collagen intertwines with the existing tendon fibers, it takes on the architecture of a normal tendon. In the final phase of healing, the collagen forms vascularized fibrous tissue, and continuity across the tear is reestablished.

Undue motion at the healing site will slow the process and, if excessive, will cause suboptimal repair. The fibrous tissue may be thinned or elongated and can result in chronic pain and an unstable joint. In a simple sprain or strain, it takes six to eight weeks for the healing to be adequate to allow normal function, and several months before the stress of exercise or sports competition can be tolerated. In most cases, resting the injury site by employing elastic wraps, splints, boots, casts, crutches and/or wheelchairs, is adequate. Depending on the joint involved and the severity of the injury, weight bearing and motion might be permitted. With other injuries, absolute rest and non-weight bearing is required.

More severe, Class 3 tears that are complete or avulsions often require surgical repair. It may require only simple suturing of the torn ends of the tendon, or reattachment of the avulsed ligament to the bone. If reattachment is not possible, tendon transfers or transplants are an option. In complex injuries, especially those that involve multiple ligaments, more extensive reconstructive surgery is necessary. Recovery from the latter takes a year and often more, and it's not uncommon for the ultimate outcome from this kind of surgery to be inadequate for the athlete to return to his or her former level of competition. Many a professional sports career has ended in this way.

When sufficient healing has occurred, rehabilitation can be very helpful in returning normal function. Motion is started as early as the injury allows. For simple sprains and strains, exercising on one's own or a few visits with a physical therapist is usually adequate. Most of the more complicated injuries and all of the surgical repairs require monitored and directed rehabilitation, in some cases, initially as an inpatient in an acute rehabilitation unit. The total time spent in rehab will be months, even a year. If you are an independently wealthy professional athlete surrounded by professional trainers, this is one kind of hardship. If you are a regular person with a job, children, and a home you care for yourself, this is a completely different kind of hardship. If you are a neurosurgeon, you think you know better than conventional wisdom and ignore it. Big mistake!

Muscle injuries follow a similar pattern. Every skeletal muscle is comprised of an organized repeating structural array of thousands of muscle fibers called myofibers bundled together by an enveloping layer of tissue called fascia. The fascia thickens into a tendon at the muscle's end, allowing for its insertion into bone. A highly specialized membrane, the sarcolemma, carries impulses from the external environment and the motor neuron into the muscle fiber, causing contraction and covers individual myofibers. On the cellular level, the myofibers are composed of myofibrils, which are themselves made up of sub-cellular myofilaments, of which there are two kinds: thin (actin) and thick (myosin). When a nerve impulse is received, calcium ion movement across the filaments' membranes creates a sliding movement of actin on myosin resulting in shortening and hence contraction of the muscle.

The repeating nature of the organization of the myofibrils in the myofilaments gives muscle both its characteristic striated appearance when seen under a microscope and its name: striated muscle.

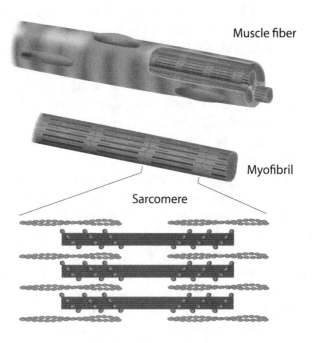

Muscle and joint anatomy.

Luckily for athletes, exercisers, and proto-humans, scattered throughout the muscle are structures called satellite cells. Some force of nature—evolution, as described initially by Charles Darwin, if you are of the scientific persuasion, intelligent design if you are not—'realized' that of all the organs in the human body, muscle is particularly prone to injury with even the most mundane of physical activity. It is, after all, possible to pull a muscle doing the everyday activities of living such as rubbing two sticks together to start a fire in your tribal cave, or lifting a leaded crystal martini glass in your man cave. Satellite cells are regenerative, unipotential adult stem cells that activate in response to muscle damage. They begin to proliferate and differentiate into myoblasts, the progenitors of muscle cells that rebuild the damaged muscle. Other organs have the ability to regenerate

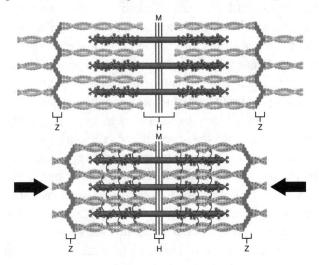

Muscle contraction.

as well, but few carry their own stem cells. Some cells, notably nerve cells, cannot regenerate at all once lost.

Evolution posits that an organism that moves by using muscle has a greater chance of surviving to reproduce if it can regenerate a damaged muscle and return to full speed running and full strength. If it can't repair the injury, its movement and strength will be degraded, making it much more likely the injured animal will become lunch for some other, uninjured animal.

At some point in time, a genetic mutation bestowed on a newborn the gene that produced satellite cells in its muscles. This allowed its injured muscles to heal more quickly shortening periods of defenselessness, and therefore allowed it to survive longer than other members of its generation. As such it gave this newly endowed creature the opportunity to mate with more of its kind. Its genetic material was passed on to the next generation, many of which also had regenerative satellite cells, allowing for longer life and more procreating and—you get the picture. Eventually all members of the species had the cells. It's an elegant and compelling theory that not only explains how proto-humans became us, but is almost universally accepted, even by some very religious people who can coexist in both the scientific and religious worlds.

If, on the other hand, you are a devotee of intelligent design, you believe that your deity came up with this idea by watching over us, seeing one of its creations with a sprained ankle not get better, become unable to catch food, become weak, and get eaten by another of its creations with good ankles. And *voila!* Unipotential adult stem cells get added to skeletal muscle to help us from becoming lunch.

Injury to muscle can occur by physical, chemical, or envenomous damage. I will describe an example of the latter in the chapter on running. Exercise causes physical injury. Muscle strain, that ubiquitous description applied to every sore muscle that ever followed a workout, is a nonspecific term that refers to the local muscle damage that comes from over-stretching the myofibers or surpassing the muscle's ability to deal with applied repetitive contractions.

Strains produce tears in the fiber structure of the muscle, the extent of which will determine how much damage is done, how much pain there will be, and how long recovery will take. Strains, pulls, tears and ruptures are essentially synonymous, but in some usage represent a continuum of severity, in the order listed, from mild to severe. In more severe injuries, the muscle tendon is also usually involved.

In the young, muscle tears are more common than tendon injuries. A young tendon is at its most elastic and will tolerate stretching without injury more than will the muscle. In the older athlete, the tendon loses some of its youthful elasticity, and tears are more likely. There will be evidence of tissue damage that includes hemorrhage, fiber disruption, and all the signs of inflammation. With time, the satellite cells activate, cellular differentiation produces new muscle, and the repair completes itself.

The time frame for repair of muscle mirrors that of ligaments and tendons. Six weeks for the mild and moderate injuries is usually sufficient, but protection of the injured muscle is as important as it is for the others. Severely torn muscles require surgical repair, with the increased recovery time and rehab that accompanies such an injury. Large tears in the fascia of the muscle allowing it to herniate through its covering sheath may also need surgery, although these are less common.

Many of us, especially me, tend to give insufficient respect to this class of injury; that is, muscle tears. They are so common and, since they are due to everyday activities as often as they are to exercise, we tend to think of them as temporary annoyances rather than the real injuries they are. If repetitive and not allowed to fully heal, they become chronic and can cause persistent pain that may never go away. I see this in my office every day, in the form of patients also coming to see me for chronic back and neck pain.

I am particularly impatient with these injuries when they occur in me. I've mentioned how bad a patient I am, and with my three significant forms of these injuries—skiing, softball and the fall from the ladder—I got back on my feet too early. Although I eventually healed, the process took longer than it needed to, and I still get an occasional twinge, particularly in the ankle. My left calf, twice injured, has never returned to its original size. It reminds me of another old saying among physicians—*Do as I say, not as I do*. When I fractured my ankle in the fall off the ladder, I had concomitant tendon injuries as well. I was the quintessential bad doctor-patient, listening patiently to what my orthopedic friends told me to do, then ignoring it and doing whatever the hell I thought was okay. I started weight bearing too quickly, converted from a boot to a simple splint too early, and took even that off before I should have. I didn't even consider physical therapy. The bone healed without incident, but I had a relapse due to delayed healing of the tendon and had to go back into the splint. Even today, nine months after the injury, I have intermittent pain and persistent swelling over the inside of my ankle. Oddly enough, it hurts more often when I'm off my feet than it does when I'm on them. Maybe I'll see a doctor about that.

"NO PAIN, NO GAIN"

This statement, ingrained in the lexicon of the exercise culture, is unquestionably the stupidest thing I have ever heard. I have heard it voiced by people who are considered experts in the field of exercise. Some of those espousing this moronic philosophy actually have degrees in this science. I am concerned they have little knowledge of injury physiology.

Pain is necessary. It is an evolutionary adaption to injury that provides the organism with necessary information about its immediate environment. It gives the organism an advantage that increases the likelihood that it will survive an adverse event, live to procreate, and pass its DNA to the next generation.

Pain makes us aware that something bad has happened. It can cause an immediate reflex action, such as the rapid muscle contraction that pulls our hand away from a hot stove. And who hasn't seen the football player writhing on the ground in agony after having his knee destroyed by a 250-pound linebacker who can run a forty-yard dash in 4.4 seconds?

If you do something physical that results in pain, that

physical activity is bad for you. It has harmed you. The pain is a sign, a huge red warning flag waving in front of your face, that the activity must be stopped, and the damage done allowed to heal. We've all done calisthenics. "Make those muscles burn!" screams the sadist on the exercise video. I don't think so. Make those muscles work, but not burn. As soon as the burn starts, STOP! Taking the workout up to, but not beyond, the point of injury makes so much more sense. Burning muscles, especially if they have been strained, have to be rested, at times treated, and even medicated. It makes it less likely that you will be able to return to that exercise when you want, and possibly, especially so for me, less likely that you will even want to return to that exercise.

Let's review.

No pain, no gain: stupid.

Yes pain, warning: stop.

No pain, much gain, assuming you are actually exercising. Exercising just to the point of muscle fatigue, but not beyond, provides great benefit. It may not be as macho as the grimacing, grunting, sweating weight lifter who is struggling to get that last possible repetition out of his body. But I suspect you'll even get in shape as quickly as the over-doer. You'll be able to work out more consistently, spend less time in the trainer's room, and less time on the disabled list requiring time off from your activity of choice.

Going beyond muscle fatigue puts the muscle into a state called anaerobic glycolysis. This is a physiologic state in which the muscle, that normally burns glucose with oxygen to provide energy, can no longer do so. Instead, the glucose is broken down without oxygen. The by-product of this form of energy production is lactic acid, which builds up in the muscle and creates that aching, failing feeling, sometimes accompanied by cramping, that we interpret as muscle fatigue.

Listen to your body. Pain is always a warning. Heed the warnings. You'll be more likely to live to procreate. And we all know how much fun procreating is.

Chapter 2

RECREATIONAL, FASHIONABLE EXERCISE: RUNNING, BICYCLING, AND YOGA

Pound, pound, pound.

Pound, pound, pound.

Imagine a garden stake you are pounding into the ground. Visualize the ten-pound sledgehammer you are using to drive that stake into the earth, and think of the force you are generating to accomplish the task. Now imagine the leg you are running on. Visualize the one-hundred-plus pound body atop the leg pounding down on top of it with every stride of a run, yard after yard, mile after mile, for hours at a time, for months or years or decades.

Pound, pound, pound.

"I'd rather be a hammer than a nail," goes the traditional song popularized by Simon and Garfunkel as 'El Condor Pasa'. Sound advice, but your leg is the nail.

Pound, pound, pound.

It's not the image the running shoe companies want you to have. But it is accurate. Again, I didn't warn you ahead of time that there would be math in this book, so I will spare you the calculations I did trying to estimate the accumulated force, in pounds per square inch, transmitted to the foot during a lifetime of running. Suffice it to say, it's a lot. Estimates of the incidence of running-related injuries vary widely, and reach as high as 79 percent. One report suggests that injuries occur in 37 to 56 percent per year of those who run regularly.[1] PER YEAR! That means the majority of runners had multiple injuries, some every year.

I suspect the truth is that the rate is over 100 percent. If you count all the minor sprains and strains that never get reported or seen for treatment, all runners have repetitive injuries. They're difficult to avoid given that the very act of running is itself repetitive. This concept is a theme I will repeat throughout this book. There are innumerable exercise- and sports- related injuries that occur every day, day in and day out.

Despite the position of the foot at the bottom of the leg and it receiving the full force of all the weight above it, the knee is actually most commonly injured by running. The foot and ankle as a unit, is in second place, followed by the hip, then in no particular order, the lower back (my turf), the muscles and their connections of the thigh, calf, and foot, the upper back and the neck (also my turf). It seems intuitive, doesn't it? All those moving parts that go into creating the motion of running, stressed repeatedly over long periods of time, finally give out.

The injuries take many forms. They can, individually or in combination, involve the ligaments, tendons, bones, cartilage, joint bursas, and nerves. In the spine, this list includes the discs. Some have exotic names like patellofemoral syndrome (runner's knee), plantar fasciitis (inflammation of the connective tissue of the muscles on the bottom of the foot), and iliotibial band syndrome (inflammation of the muscle fascia along the outside of the knee). There is a common final pathway for most of these injuries—inflammation. With the exception of fractures, most of the other injuries involve soft tissues of one or more types that react to the stretching, pulling, twisting, bending, and pounding by becoming inflamed. The nerves that serve these tissues react by creating pain, a seemingly annoying but absolutely necessary bodily defense mechanism that we have seen lets us know there is a problem that needs repair.

With time, as repetitive injury and inflammation take their toll, there is degeneration of the structures involved, and chronic pain and dysfunction set in. At that point, inflammation often isn't the problem and healing isn't possible; the tissue is worn out, irreversibly altered and anatomically changed. Treatment is directed at symptom management rather than rehabilitation. When a joint is involved and an end stage is reached, joint replacement is an option if non-surgical treatments can't control pain.

The injuries I outline above are only the 'regular' everyday injuries sustained by runners. There are also the more unusual hazards of the sport. Running in a field exposes one to the irregularities of the terrain, with a turned ankle or the ominous 'boot top' fracture a possibility. The latter is a fracture above the ankle, seen in skiers at the top of the boot that can occur when a runner encounters a hole in the ground. And if we're talking fully informed consent, I might remind you that when running outside, dogs can bite you, cars can run over you, and there is even the rare but reported lightning strike! We can add sunburn, chafing, smog inhalation, road rash from falls, dehydration, shin splints, side stitches, bug and snakebites, and the "loneliness of long distance running" to the list as well.

But to step away for a moment from the more esoteric possibilities and get back to the basic injuries that come from running: the majority of treatments for these injuries are anti-inflammatory. Rest stops the injuring event, aided when necessary by wrapping, bracing, or casting. Elevation and ice reduce the swelling. Ice is also an analgesic. Anti-inflammatory medications reduce pain and slow the inflammatory response itself. Steroids, both ingested and injected, are the strongest of this class of drug.

Physical therapy is universally used for a lingering injury. It helps with the actual healing of the injury once the initial inflammatory phase has passed by stretching, toning and building muscle, reconditioning tendons and ligaments, and returning normal range of motion to joints.

In some cases, surgery is necessary. If so, it is the rare athlete who returns to his or her former peak performance. We all know a high school or college athlete, and have read about pros, whose sports career ended after knee surgery or a back operation. Even the casual exerciser often has difficulty returning to former exercise levels after a serious injury.

A wise heart surgeon with whom I interned told me that the best way to avoid problems in his post-operative patients was to anticipate them. The best way to treat an injury is similar. Anticipate it and avoid it. You could do what my father, of blessed memory, told me to do. "Every time I get the urge to exercise," he told me, "I lie down until the urge goes away." Dad got his exercise acting as pallbearer for his friends who exercised. That is, he was possibly a bit too sedentary. (That is, until his first heart attack. After that he rode a stationary bike every day he wasn't carrying a casket.)

Wearing a good running shoe is a start. Unfortunately, they have become ridiculously expensive, and come in so many models and styles, it's difficult to know if they really deliver the protection and performance enhancement they claim. I suspect they don't. But if you are fortunate enough to inherit a silver mine, go to the mall and find a pair that fit well and are comfortable. And if you run frequently, buy new ones more often than average. They do wear out, just like us.

If possible, run on a soft surface. Many runners use the roads. They are convenient, go everywhere, are often scenic, are free (not counting local taxes), and can usually be found at your front door. But asphalt is hard, hot in the summer, and slippery in bad weather. The 'pound index,' a term I just made up, is the highest.

Pound, pound, pound.

Tracks at athletic fields are often made of a composite material and have more give, reducing the pound index. They are harder to find, and at times not available if they are otherwise engaged by a competitive event or school usage. Fields and other natural surfaces are softer still, but I've already discussed the hidden dangers lurking there.

Indoor surfaces, if synthetic, are generally softer. They also keep one out of harm's way associated with the great outdoors. However, they cost money. If it is at a gym or spa, there are membership fees. If you use a treadmill at home, you have to buy it. It's also boring in the extreme. You can listen to music, watch television, read, or let your mind wander. But it's not like jogging through the Grand Tetons, or past Grand Central Station. The purists I know will have none of the indoor variety. Indoor tracks made of hardwood look great, but have a high pound index, and get slippery with sweat. And did I mention that they're boring?

Some will say that what follows is a cheap shot, but there is no end to the number of publications extolling the salutary effects of exercise. Examples of the opposite are fair game.

Jim Fixx was a celebrated athlete and author. In 1977 he wrote *The Complete Book of Running* and is credited with popularizing both the sport of running and furthering the general interest in fitness that was growing quickly at the time. In 1984, at the age of fifty-two, he died suddenly of a heart attack after a run.

Ironically, his book *Maximum Sports Performance* was published after his death. It extolled the great physical and psychological benefits of sports in general and running in particular.

His autopsy revealed advanced coronary artery disease. He had a strong family history: his father died at forty-three, also of a heart attack. The prevailing wisdom was that Fixx would have died even earlier if he hadn't been a runner. That's one explanation. After all, when he started running at age thirty-five, he weighed 240 pounds, and smoked. When he died seventeen years later, he was 60 pounds lighter and a non-smoker.

Another one, also plausible, is that if he hadn't stressed his heart as aggressively as he did, he might still be alive. I am of the belief that there is a proper medium between being completely sedentary and fanatically active. There is no one place on that spectrum that works for everyone. You will have to find it for yourself. Keep in mind what I said about pain. That's especially true if it's chest pain.

There's another old joke that says we only get so many heartbeats in life. The faster your heart rate, the sooner you use them up. On the other hand, the better shape you are in, the slower your resting heart rate will be. So maybe it's a wash. Losing weight and quitting smoking have unequivocal health benefits. No amount of digging will reveal evidence to the contrary, and I don't even have a joke to refute it.

But is there a level of physical activity that is counter-productive to good health? Unquestionably. I wish I knew what the level is. It's clearly different for each of us. Like many situations, retrospective sight is 20/20. Once you reach a point of exercise that produces pain or injury, you have clearly found your level. Unfortunately, if the first sign is sudden death, there is no resetting it.

John "Jack" Kelly was the scion of a wealthy and famous Philadelphia family. He was the brother of actress Grace Kelly, later the Princess of Monaco, and the son of an Olympic gold medalist. He was famous in his own right as an oarsman and participated in four Olympics in Crew, winning the bronze medal at the 1956 Summer Olympics in Melbourne. In 1947, he won the James E. Sullivan award as the top US amateur athlete.

Kelly was a storied athlete. In addition to the above awards, he managed the gold medal eight-man scull at the 1964 summer games in Tokyo. In 1970, he became the president of the Amateur Athletic Union and president of the United States Olympic Committee in 1985.

He was a regular on "Boathouse Row," the iconic Tudor homes along the Schuylkill River just upstream from the Philadelphia Art Museum where the local rowing community and universities house their sculls. The outlines of the homes are adorned with white lights that are turned on every night, creating a unique and artistic scene that has become a signature of the city. Kelly could often be seen on an oar in the early morning hours, and was instrumental in popularizing the sport of crew.

In the Philadelphia media, and by reputation, he was portrayed as a paragon of the physically fit adult who worked hard to keep himself in enviable shape. Possibly, he worked a little too hard. In 1985, at the age of fifty-seven, he died after jogging to the Philadelphia Athletic Club. Earlier that day, he had been rowing. His autopsy confirmed, just as with Jim Fixx, the presence of coronary artery disease. And just as Fixx did, Kelly exercised in the extreme.

Both these tragic deaths, occurring a year apart, happened at a time that predates many of the cholesterol-lowering and cardiac protective drugs that exist today. It's possible that if these two world-class athletes had been taking them, the cardiac stress that led to their deaths might have been better tolerated, and non-fatal. However,

these are not isolated events, just among the more celebrated ones. They continue to happen on a regular basis,
and represent only a small but attention-grabbing fraction
of the total number of injuries that result from running.

Dr. Geoffrey Temple is a family physician, and a colleague and referring doctor of mine. He is also a neighbor
and friend. I had dinner with his wife Andrea and him the
evening before I wrote this passage. He is an avid jogger
and in good shape for his fifty-four years. His story is one
of the more unusual ones in my file of jogging injuries and
attests to the myriad of possible negative consequences of
exercise.

Across the street from Geoff's home is a large field,
part of a land preserve that is used recreationally by many
people. A few months earlier, while jogging through the
field, he felt something bite or sting him on the side of
his calf. He reacted, as do we all, with his hand, brushing
at the site of the pain. To this day, he's not entirely sure
what it was.

Later that evening, the bite began to swell and became
increasingly painful. Over the next few days, he developed
a fever to 103 degrees Fahrenheit and thought, diagnosing
himself as many doctors are wont to do, that the growing lesion was infected. Suspecting methicillin-resistant
Staphylococcus aureus (MRSA), he put himself on antibiotics, with no improvement. With the fever, swelling,
and pain unabated, he went to the emergency room. Suspecting an abscess, a surgeon opened the now egg-sized
lump, but there was no pus. The biopsy of the excised
tissue showed no infection, rather vasculitis, a hallmark
of inflammation, and necrosis, dead tissue. Before the

bite/sting finally cleared up, it required a second, larger operation to excise more necrotic skin and muscle. At one point, when things seemed to be at their worst, Geoff actually thought he might lose part or all of his leg.

Venom experts were consulted, but the exact diagnosis was never confirmed. No one was familiar with a stinging insect that could produce this exaggerated a response, and the site of the bite, high up on the calf just below the knee, is an unlikely place for a snake strike. Additionally, venomous snakes are rare in our area.

This particular story has a happy ending. The wound has healed completely, and Geoff is back out in the field jogging, with some trepidation. It's a stretch, I admit, to label this as an exercise-induced injury. It happened, however, because he was outside running. If Mother Nature has it in for you, she can give you the all-time mother of oddball injuries; just ask Geoff. I listed a variety of possible things that can happen to someone running outdoors. Although I listed a lightning strike as a possibility, it never occurred to me that venom should be on that list until I heard Geoff's story. I expect the likelihood of such an injury is even less than that of getting hit by lightning. So I told Geoff that he should at all costs avoid running in a thunderstorm. I've seen people electrocuted by lightning. It is awful.

Pound, pound, pound.

BICYCLING

Bicycling is a sport I tried to get into. There is a group of doctors at my hospital who are serious about it and often ride together. Several of them are advanced riders, and one of them, German by birth, actually rode for the German national team in his youth. It was riding with them that I sustained the wrist fracture I described in the Introduction.

As road cycling and mountain biking have become more popular, the number of injuries related to these activities has increased. Decalzi and associates, writing in the journal *Orthopedics* in April 2013, looked at the epidemiology of this phenomenon in a competitive road cycling team in Los Angeles. The authors also reviewed the literature of sports injuries.

The team's approximately three hundred members were queried by email and questioned on several metrics: years of experience riding, mileage, training and race activities, and crashes. The response rate was low. Twenty-nine, or 10 percent, answered the questionnaire. Among the twenty-nine respondents, there were 121 crashes, an average of 4.2 crashes per rider.[2] The results' meaning must be seen within the limitations of this study. The small response rate may inject an element of selection bias and not reflect the experience of the entire racing club. Additionally, it is a prevalence study, not an incidence evaluation, which makes it difficult to compare this to other studies. The respondents however, do represent an average of fourteen years of riding experience and more than four crashes per individual.[3] This high rate of injury dovetails with the results of other investigators.

Quoting other studies, Decalzi introduces his study with the statistics of cycling injuries. According to the United States Consumer Safety Products Commission, in 2009, there were an estimated 554,000 bicycle injuries. Among children, 300,000 injuries produced 15,000 inpatient hospital stays,[4] making bicycle riding, among common participation sports, the one with the highest absolute number of injuries.[5] The injuries range from the minor—falls producing abrasions and lacerations—to the major—high speed crashes causing serious head injuries, multiple-trauma and death. Chronic non-traumatic injuries are also common, due to both overuse and bicycling position. Tendonitis, muscle and joint pain commonly result from the repetitive nature of cycling movements. Compression neuropathy of the median and ulnar nerves in the hand and the pudendal nerve in the groin come from body positions necessary for bicycle riding. Cervical pain is associated with the neck extension created by the head-up position necessary to maintain forward vision. The cost of treating cycling- related acute traumatic injury from U.S. data in 2000 was estimated to be $8 billion.[6] Conn, et al., in an incidence study, looked at the rate of injuries requiring formal medical attention per 1,000 population of individuals participating in common sporting activities.[7] Cycling was second on a cumulative basis, with 2.6 injuries per 1,000, behind basketball at 3.9 injuries per 1,000.

Cycling is a sport that confers many physical and psychological benefits, but not without potential cost. It is a high speed sport, performed on hard or irregular terrain, with many potential ways to create injury and with little body protection. I will look at some of these injuries in more detail.

Despite information like this, of which I was then as now all too aware, I really did try to get into cycling. I bought a good bike, an aluminum Trek that was light-weight and high tech with lots of gears. The derailleur (the device that changes the gear) operated from mechanisms in the brake handles, an option I didn't even know existed since the last bike I bought was prehistoric compared to this one. I bought it at a bicycle specialty shop owned by a former professional racer. It was ordered according to the specifications of my body dimensions and assembled after I was measured in more ways than I thought it was possible to measure the human body. The seat and handlebars were positioned and their height adjusted according to specific angles I was supposed to maintain to improve the efficiency of my riding.

Despite spending what I thought was an absurd amount of money on the thing, I was shocked to realize that I had purchased a fairly pedestrian road bike. The top of the line carbon fiber Italian models sold for five figures, as much as you might spend for a new car!

And don't forget the clothing. Wearing gym shorts and cotton tee shirts just doesn't work. Not only do you look out of place with your riding companions, but the material is not designed to help you evaporate the sweat that accumulates in surprisingly large amounts when riding, especially in the summer. Bike shorts and jerseys are made of micro polyester, a synthetic fiber that is very lightweight and wicks the sweat away from the skin surface into the fabric and speeds evaporation. The first time I rode with my doctor friends was before I made the investment. I had an old off-road bike with wide tires, and cotton clothing that absorbed rather than wicked the sweat. Midway through the ride I had about ten pounds of moisture saturating my shirt and shorts that not only added weight but also blocked the way for any additional perspiration to escape my skin surface. I was drenched.

Bicycle shorts are their own story. Made of the same lightweight micropolyester material, they have a special adaption that helps with the discomfort of riding with your ischial tuberosities (those bones deep in your butt) perched on a narrow seat for hours at a time. A good seat is made of a gel material, and so are the pads sewn into the shorts. I was taken aback however, when the shop owner, from whom I bought all this paraphernalia, explained that the shorts worked best when riding "Scotsman" style; that is, with nothing under the kilt. Wearing underwear adds an additional surface between your skin and the gel pads that creates friction and adds rubbing, and goodness knows no one wants added rubbing on their ischial tuberosities.

Then there is the helmet. This is a serious piece of equipment for bicyclists, and although it does not render the rider invulnerable, as I will describe shortly, it is essential, and is the single most important purchase that comes with outfitting yourself for riding, regardless of the surface on which you ride. I bought the best one the shop sold. It's made of lightweight, high grade, strong, impact-resistant plastic. It has replaceable padding inside and adjustable straps to facilitate a comfortable fit. It is sleek and aerodynamic. It even has a short visor to shield your eyes, and in my case remind me which side is the front since it is remarkably symmetric along its long axis.

A peculiar characteristic of this clothing is its design. The colors are varied, vivid, and loud. There is all manner of shapes, pictures, crests, writing, and color mixing that dazzles the eye. If you watch the Tour de France, you've seen this. Teams will all wear the same outfits that help identify them and distinguish them from other riding teams. They spend a lot to have them created by famous clothing designers.

There is, however, another important benefit to the resultant look; it is highly visible. Riding on public streets requires one to share the road with cars, and it is a distinct disadvantage to be invisible to drivers. Although more and more, I am seeing roadways with specific bicycle lanes lined off at their sides, I still want to be clearly seen by every driver who approaches me from the rear. Who knows if that driver, looking at the narrow lanes with the big bicycle and rider stenciled on the asphalt surface, understands that it's for riders like me and not for the two wheels on the right side of his car. Not everyone is a clear thinker. And remember that part about surviving to procreate?

The first time I put on my outfit, I thought I looked ridiculous. Skintight shorts, a waist-length jersey that showed my slightly protuberant belly, and a helmet, despite being designed by experts, sitting on top of my head, above my ears, looking like the cap of a mushroom, I ventured forth to meet my like-dressed co-riders.

All this equipment comes with its own hefty price tag. Buy a good helmet, a few changes of clothing, good shoes, a riding computer for the handlebars, a pouch for under the seat, a small, portable tire pump, and a water bottle holder or two, and you've spent another four-figure sum. Add in a bike rack for the car, a high volume tire pump, gloves, sports glasses, a rear view mirror; I could go on forever. You get the picture. Ka-ching, ka-ching, ka-ching.

My wife was fully on board with my decision to start riding, realizing that with my aversion to exercise, anything I did that got me more active was a good thing. The price tag was worth it, she figured. It was in that first summer of riding, when I was just starting to get in better shape and feel that I could keep up with my more experienced riding partners, that I encountered the road shoulder that I carelessly drifted onto in a moment of lapsed attention. I've already described the wrist fracture that resulted (without falling, remember). What I didn't tell you was the psychological fallout of that injury.

I am not a youngster and, although already in the latter stage of my career when the accident happened, I was not contemplating retirement. I was still helping to support my adult children, who were struggling in the early stages of their careers. My youngest was about to start college, and with tuition bills looming, having grossly underestimated the amount of money I needed to save for college when she was born, I couldn't afford to retire. My knowledge of the havoc that a scaphoid bone fracture can wreak on a surgeon's career terrified me. It also brought back memories of my friend, Kim Marsh.

Kim is a neurosurgeon too. There are several that make it into this book. Kim and I trained together at Penn. He was one year ahead of me in the residency program. Several years ago Kim came to visit Pam and me in our home. He looked tan and healthy. The color came from his new career as a charter boat captain, which he took up as a necessity after a hand injury ended his surgery career. While playing softball, he caught a fly ball with his bare right hand, his dominant hand. It shattered several of the hand's small delicate bones, and required several operations to try and fix. He never went back into the operating room again. He did land on his feet, however, and actually seemed happy. He certainly had one of the best tans I ever saw.

I, however, have no marketable skills other than medicine. I know nothing about seafaring and get queasy in small boats on anything other than calm seas, a leftover from a case of malignant seasickness I had while marlin fishing with my father as a young boy. As I write this, I don't really know if I have any future as a writer. So I found absolutely no humor in my wrist fracture and the real possibility that it could be a career killer. Even though Bob Takei, my hand surgeon, stressed the more likely good outcome, he did say the real result sometimes could take a year to know. I was feeling pretty good at a month, and already back in the OR, but that yearlong timetable played with my head.

Needless to say, my biking activities came to a screeching halt. After a few months, when I felt reasonably sure that I was not going to be one of the fracture-healing failures, I went for an easy ride on a flat trail along the Schuylkill River. This time I did fall. Remember the expensive riding shoes I briefly mentioned above? They have a specific design that includes a cleat in the bottom of the shoe that locks your foot into the pedal. This allows for increased efficiency of riding in that you can both pull up on the pedal with one leg while pushing down with the other one. It takes some getting used to however, and, although it is easy to quickly release your foot from the pedal, there are times, experienced by all riders, where your foot seems to get stuck. When you're coming to a stop, it's a bad time for that to happen. You see where this is going. Sure enough, on that first ride after getting back on the bike, I had just such a fall. The tendency in that situation is to extend your arm to break your fall. There's no thinking about it. It's a reflex protective motion. As luck would have it, I fell to the side away from my healing wrist, at an almost complete stop, and, although I fell full force on my extended hand and arm, I escaped uninjured, pride not included.

I stayed off the bike for all of the last two years. Just this summer, I decided to remount. Every summer, my family vacations for two weeks in Stone Harbor, New Jersey, on the famous Jersey Shore. Stone Harbor is one of a string of barrier islands, separated from the mainland by a series of bays that run along the New Jersey coastline, from Sandy Hook in the north, near New York, to Cape May at the southern tip of the state. These islands vary in width, being only a few hundred feet wide in some places. You can travel the length of the islands using the bridges that connect them together at their northern and southern ends, but driving through the towns on the islands is slow going due to stop lights and signs, and the ever-present twenty-five-miles-per-hour speed limit. If you want to travel any distance, most travelers take the causeway that links each island to the mainland and connects to the

Garden State Parkway, a high-speed road that runs north and south the length of the state.

The island roads and their connector bridges are, however, pleasant roads to bike on. They're flat, with the exception of the bridges, and picturesque, especially away from each island's centrally located town center.

The road that runs south out of Stone Harbor is narrow and winds gently through the surrounding wetlands that come up to the road's very edge. Its two lanes meander through the grassy, sandy terrain teeming with the wildlife unique to this protected habitat. Graceful cranes, terns, and gulls float above, occasionally diving for the prey that lives hidden in the marsh grass. The reeds blend into the sea and sway in the wind swirls that dance off the ocean waves, giving the illusion of continuity of land and water.

The island tapers here and disappears into the ocean inlet that joins to the back bays, separating Stone Harbor from Wildwood, New Jersey, to the south. It was on these roads that I reentered the world of bicycling. That the roads were mostly flat was an advantage for me, since I was completely out of shape. The challenge comes from the winds that are ever-present on these islands. Although they are a pleasant break from the summer heat, they can be as hard as a steep hill to bike through. When they're at your back, you feel like a pro. When they're in your face, it's a struggle.

Stone Harbor and Avalon are on the same island, known as Seven Mile Island. Any guess how long it is? I used to think Stone Harbor was an odd name for a town that had neither stone nor a harbor. I have subsequently learned, from the town's museum docent, that a Captain Stone who became stranded in the barrier island's inlet channel during a storm in the early nineteenth century bestowed the name. Riding from my house to each end of the island and back to the house is a nice fourteen-mile circuit, not a long ride for a veteran, but fine for the novice. It is my usual route, although on days when I feel unusually energized, I'll go further and cross the bridges to the neighboring islands. One of my rides was a twenty-five-mile ride inland where the winds are less of a factor, but the temperature is usually higher. My personal best, before the wrist injury, was thirty-two miles.

I had planned to ride every day. In my two weeks there this past July, I rode four times. It's a start. One could say the abbreviated schedule was due to the psychic trauma of my broken wrist, my fear of being out of work, and the grim story (with the happy ending) of Kim Marsh. It's closer to the truth to say I didn't ride every day because I'm lazy. Although the "danger in exercise" theme of this book is always in my mind, my aversion to exercise is equally rooted in my enjoyment of lassitude. Maybe if I stayed with it and finally reached that hoped- for but elusive endorphin high, I would be driven back to the bike, unable to deny myself the endogenous drug effect produced by repetitively pushing your body to the limits of tolerance.

Until that day, I'll proceed cautiously. I have a new rule. When I ride, I pre-dial my GPS enabled cell phone to 911, and keep it within easy reach. That way, if I get hit by a car, or have a heart attack on a remote road, and I'm just a little lucky, I'll have a brief period in which I can retrieve the phone and hit the call button before I lapse into a coma. The police, I would hope, will know to access the GPS signal and come find me. So far, so good for me. Not so for some others.

The wheel is the consensus choice for the most important invention in the history of the world, having done more to influence the progress of human civilization than any other invention.[8] I agree. It is part of our lives in innumerable ways, both for good and for bad. The internal combustion engine attached to either two or four of them accounted for thirty-seven thousand fatalities in the United States in 2012.[9] The two-wheeled version powered by the human leg has its share of sad stories as well. Fred Epstein was an internationally recognized pediatric neurosurgeon from New York City, at New York University, and later became the founding director of the Institute for Neurology and Neurosurgery at the Beth Israel Medical Center. He was a celebrated surgeon and a wonderful person.

I had the privilege of meeting him on several occasions during the time I was training at the Children's Hospital of Philadelphia. Dr. Epstein was a good friend of my chief, Luis Schut. Both of them were among the founders of Pediatric Neurosurgery as a subspecialty of neurosurgery and each developed training programs, from which I and many other residents had the good fortune to benefit. His academic interest was in tumors of the central nervous system. At the height of his career, he had what was probably the world's most extensive experience with removing tumors from the spinal cord, and neurosurgeons from all over the world came to New York to learn from him.

He was an enthusiastic and experienced cyclist, riding several times a week near his home in Greenwich, Connecticut. Fifteen miles was a common distance for him. On Sunday September 30, 2001, his bike hit a rut in the road, throwing him forward over the handlebars. He landed on his head, and, despite wearing a helmet, which he did conscientiously, he sustained a severe closed head injury. He was taken to Stamford Hospital where a CT scan revealed a skull fracture and an acute subdural hematoma: a blood clot layered over the surface of the brain. Dr. Epstein was in a coma from the injury and the pressure being placed on his brain from the hematoma. An emergency craniotomy was performed to remove the blood clot and repair the damage that was causing the bleeding.

After this kind of surgery, it is difficult to know what the outcome will be. It is dependent on the severity of the injury and what, if any, additional injury becomes apparent in the hours after the initial one. The prognosis can at times be suggested by the patient's condition at the time of arrival to the hospital, and he arrived unconscious.

His coma lasted a month. When Dr. Epstein finally awakened, his mental status and personality slowly returned, and by the time he was transferred to Mount Sinai Medical Center Rehabilitation service in late October, he was able to recognize people he knew from before the accident. With time, his cognitive abilities returned to near-normal.

Unfortunately, his physical abilities did not. He suffered partial paralysis on his right side, and double vision. He was often seen wearing an eye patch as a result. He was never able to return to the operating room, and a giant talent was lost to neurosurgery.

He died on July 9, 2006, although not of causes related to his injury. He had developed malignant melanoma, the most virulent of the skin cancers and died of metastatic disease.[10]

In the ying and yang of the bicycle world, that which can be both good and bad, Herb Auerbach serves as a clear example. Herb is the chairman of the Department of Pathology at my hospital. He credits biking with getting his weight to the perfect place for his body frame and putting him into the best shape he's ever been in. He is one of the stronger riders in the group of doctors who bike together, the group I used to ride with and someday plan to rejoin, maybe. Last year, the group was riding in Bucks County, a semi-rural suburb of Philadelphia with narrow roads, lots of hills, and drivers that generally respect cyclists. It is dotted with covered bridges that cross the many streams and small rivers in the county.

On a bright day, when you enter one of these bridges, the transition from bright light to covered shade causes a momentary darkening of vision, lasting until your pupils dilate in the reduced light. In addition, these bridges are usually at the bottom of a hill since water is usually at geographic low points. Herb, as he often does, had ridden ahead of the group. He goes for a while, and then doubles back and rejoins the pack. On this day, he was ahead, out of sight of his companions, when he rode through a covered bridge at a good clip, since he was coming off a hill. In the instant when his vision was dimmed, he came upon two women who were walking through the bridge from the opposite direction. At the last second, he saw them, swerved to avoid them, and crashed.

His helmet cracked, as did several ribs, his lower lip, and a few teeth. In addition there were a variety of contusions, lacerations, and abrasions, the common triad of injuries to a body in motion making contact with a stationary hard surface, sometimes known as road rash. The other riders, all physicians, caught up with him shortly after the accident. Among them was Stan Silverman, a senior member of the critical care team at the hospital. Herb was briefly unconscious and still confused when first seen, and Stan immediately recognized what was likely a serious head injury.

The 911 emergency system was activated, and Herb was transported to our hospital where he was admitted to the Emergency Trauma Center as a Trauma Alert, a hospital-wide alert system that activates a designated team of physicians, nurses, respiratory, laboratory, and radiology technicians, chaplains and social workers. I was on-call for neurosurgery that day.

Most of his visible injuries were superficial and not serious. The chest x-ray however, revealed a pneumothorax. One of his broken ribs had punctured a lung causing it to collapse. A chest tube was immediately inserted and attached to suction in order to re-expand the lung.

Once stable, he was taken for a CT scan, which showed multiple cerebral hemorrhagic contusions. This was similar to the injury sustained by Dr. Epstein, but without the large collection of blood compressing the brain from the surface.

A repeat scan six hours later showed the contusions had

enlarged, but they stabilized on subsequent scans. Herb spent four days in the Intensive Care Unit. His mental status waxed and waned for several days, but with gradual and steady improvement went back to normal. The head injury did not require surgery, and he never needed an intracranial pressure monitor as he was never in a coma. His wife Lisa, also a physician and a close friend of my wife Pam, hovered nearby throughout the scary ordeal. Although this kind of injury can leave permanent damage, Herb escaped with a full recovery. He is, however, as with all brain injuries, more prone to a future injury, should one occur, being more serious and long-lasting.

It hasn't seemed to affect Herb. He got right back up in the saddle and returned to serious riding as soon as he could, much sooner than most of us taking care of him wanted. He clearly has a more resilient psyche than do I. I retreated from a wrist fracture. Herb steamed right through a serious head injury. So in order to defend my psychological strength, I reiterate, I'm lazy.

What is the point of all these bicycling horror stories? Am I trying to scare you? You betcha, as they say in Alaska. I don't want and don't really need to enumerate the healthy benefits of bicycling. They are obvious and well known to exercise enthusiasts. The rest of us can figure them out, too. Nor do I want to reiterate the routine musculoskeletal injuries that are common to cycling. I've already described them in the chapter on running, and they are essentially the same; sprains, strains, etc.

Bicycle riding is different from running. It is a high-speed sport, using a vehicle that provides absolutely no protection. It's really no different than riding a motorcycle, except the speeds are slower, and we all know how dangerous motorcycles are. Neurosurgeons call them "donorcycles" because when death results from a motorcycle head injury, it can be a great source of donor organs. Strong riders can routinely maintain speeds of twenty to twenty-five miles per hour and reach beyond forty miles per hour downhill. Falling at that speed can cause serious injury as the examples clearly show. No amount of caution and preparation can ensure an accident won't happen. Loose gravel, broken glass, inconsiderate drivers, a change in lighting, wet and uneven surfaces, and a hundred other potential hazards can cause an accident. The best helmet can sometimes fail, and even when it doesn't, it can't always protect the brain from the kind of blow that will cause the brain to impact the inner table of the skull. No other part of the body has any protection at all. Fractures and dislocations are common.

There are ways to reduce risk. Take care of your equipment. Have your bike checked regularly by someone who knows what he or she is doing. Keep the gears and chain clean and lubricated. Make sure the derailleurs are working properly so the gears change when you want them to. Inspect your tires for weak spots. Nothing will cause a fall faster than a blowout. Wear proper clothing regardless of how ostentatious it looks. My making fun of it doesn't negate the fact that it really does make a difference. Have a good quality helmet. I'll say that again: get a good quality helmet. A serious head injury can change your life forever. I've seen it more times than I care to remember. Stay off busy roads as much as possible. Drive your bike to the back roads where traffic is thin and drivers expect to see bicyclists. Ride with others. Although my trick of pre-dialing your cell phone is a hedge, riding in a group allows for immediate help if you are injured, so ride with friends. One of the advantages of being a doctor is that many of my friends are doctors too. When I ride with friends, it's likely that at least some of them will be physicians. If possible, make friends with doctors and ride with a senior member of a critical care team like Herb did. You can't be too careful.

Sometimes it's just a matter of the stars aligning in the right way. Stan's presence may have saved Herb's life. If he had been riding alone, he might have died.

Finally, and most importantly, stay alert. I always tell my residents, as I was taught years ago, that the best way to avoid trouble with a patient is to anticipate it. Know what can go wrong and look for it before it finds you. The same can be said for bicycling. Pay attention to what's around you, especially traffic. Keep your eye on the road surface and adjust speed and course when necessary. Look around bends in the road to see what's ahead as soon as possible. Be aware of sudden changes in light levels. Anticipate unseen obstacles appearing suddenly in places where your vision is obscured. Remember my momentary lapse of concentration and its result. Many riders listen to music or other MP3 offerings. That's OK as long as you don't allow yourself to become lulled. Vigilance is essential. STAY ALERT!

So why do I ride? Well at present, I don't, although I'm slowly getting back into it. But it is fun. Also, I already mentioned the bit of a gut I have showing under my biking jersey. Riding is a great way to lose weight and keep it off if you ride regularly. On one ride with Herb, we biked to New Hope, a small village on the river known for its art galleries, small restaurants and bakery shops. We stopped at one of them and had a pastry that had at least as many calories as I was going to burn on the ride, but at least there was no guilt.

On cool days, riding is an absolute pleasure. It's also a great way to get to know the back byways and roads less traveled near where you live. In the fall, when the leaves are turning colors, it's spectacular, especially on the scenic roads of Pennsylvania's Bucks County with its rolling hills, canals, and Delaware River valley. Just remember, Autumn leaves are beautiful, but they fall into the road and get wet. Beauty can be a beast. Be aware, and ride safely.

YOGA

My niece Katie has recently returned from two months in India where she studied with renowned masters of the art of yoga. She is a tall, statuesque member of the Millennial generation in her thirties. She lives in Manhattan where she works in the fashion industry in design and marketing. It seems almost cliché to say that a young health-conscious woman working in a trendy urban profession practices yoga. Of course she does. She not only practices but, as mentioned, teaches too. I really tried to resist saying she practices what she preaches, but preach is exactly what she did at a recent family gathering. I told her I was working on a book that included a segment on the dangers associated with yoga. She became as testy as I've ever seen her, and I've known her all her life.

Despite my trying to explain the intent of the book, she became defensive and put me in the same category as the author of a recent *New York Times* article, William J. Broad. A forty-year practitioner of yoga, he wrote *The Science of Yoga: The Risks and Rewards*, published in February 2012. The book is a very positive and optimistic look at the practice of yoga. One chapter, however, dwells on its dangers, and Broad, a *Times* writer and two-time Pulitzer Prize winner, excerpted it in an article in the newspaper entitled *How Yoga Can Wreck Your Body*. The article caught the attention of the yoga community and many, like Katie, thought it was an unfair focus on the small negative part of yoga, eclipsing the great benefits it offers. The article was published in January 2012, a month before the book was released, so few knew that it was part of an otherwise yoga-friendly treatment.

Katie thought I was going to do the same thing, and she was entirely correct. But I never got the chance to tell her why: that I am telling the little-heard other side of exercise; she was that angry with her uncle. Maybe she'll read the book and see what she didn't let me tell her.

I never did find out if she's had any yoga-related injuries. She avoided me for the rest of the day, joining me only in group conversations having nothing to do with exercise. I think I've replaced my brother-in-law as the bad uncle.

Broad, in his *Times* article, discusses not only the injuries typically associated with yoga, but also the reasons they occur, and therefore how they can be avoided, or at least lessened. He also describes a serious group of injuries involving the blood supply to the brain and resulting in stroke. He uses Glenn Black as his guide through this controversial corner of yoga. Black is well known within the yoga community. When Broad sought him out in 2009, Black had been teaching for almost forty years. He had a reputation for helping those with yoga- related injuries rehabilitate by using a more measured style of yoga.

Years earlier, Broad had herniated a lumbar intervertebral disk and had developed a yoga routine that kept his pain at bay. Then in 2007, while doing a pose touted as restorative of health, his back, as he describes it, "gave way. With it went my belief, naïve in retrospect, that yoga was a source only of healing and never harm."[11] Black, he surmised, given his reputation, could yoga him back to health. What Black told him could have been taken from this book. Give up yoga, he said. "It's simply too likely to cause harm."

Black believes, as I do, that the naïveté Broad discovered he labored under afflicts the majority of yoga practitioners. I of course believe that almost everyone who engages in exercise and sport for its health benefits is unaware of, or at least inattentive to, the inherent dangers of participation. "Not just students but celebrated teachers too, Black said [to Broad], injure themselves in droves because most have underlying physical weaknesses or problems that make serious injury all but inevitable."

The same could be said for any exercise routine, although yoga carries the aura of being a healing art. Not so, says Black, who feels yoga is for those who are physically fit. Teaching it to a large group of people in variable physical condition, and with disparate past medical histories, invites injury. There is no "one size fits all" in yoga. He believes it can be used therapeutically, but the teacher must know the pupil. Black therefore endeavors to know those he teaches and to determine those poses and positions they should avoid. Although Black studied with a prominent physical therapist who developed treatment regimens specific for the musculoskeletal problems of actors and dancers, he does not profess to have formal training in matching yoga exercises to the various injuries his students have. In place of training he has forty years of experience.

Black is not alone in his concern about the dangers inherent in yoga. The International Association of Yoga Therapists (IAYT) publishes the *International Journal of Yoga Therapy*. In 2008 it included an article by Jani Mikkonen and others entitled "A Survey of Musculoskeletal Injuries among *Ashtanga Vinyasa* Yoga Practitioners." Three hundred yoga practitioners in two centers in Finland were queried about their history. The authors were blinded to the individuals' personal experiences and didn't know who, if any, of those receiving the questionnaire had ever been injured. One hundred and ten, or 37 percent, returned completed questionnaires.

The primary objectives of the study were to determine the proportion of injuries and the injury rate per one thousand hours of participation. Secondary objectives were to elucidate the location, type and outcome of the injuries.

Of the 110 answering, 68 reported having at least one injury lasting one month or longer, for an injury rate of 62 percent. A total of 107 musculoskeletal injuries were reported indicating multiple injuries in a subset of the respondents. The rate of first injuries was 1.18 per one thousand hours of practice. If reoccurrence of pre-existing injuries and low back pain were included, the rate rose to 1.45 injuries per one thousand hours. In addition to the lower back, lower extremity injuries of the hamstring muscle and the knee were the most common injury sites. None of those injured considered their injury to have caused permanent impairment.

No one is immune, including the teachers. Black relates that he knows instructors with such bad back problems they teach lying down. Broad faults some of the giants of yoga with failing to include this darker side of its practice while extolling the benefits. "They celebrate its ability to calm, cure, energize and strengthen. Yoga can lower your blood pressure, make chemicals that act as antidepressants, even improve your sex life. But the yoga community long remained silent about its potential to inflict blinding pain."[12] Three of yoga's modern gurus, Jagannath G. Gune in his 1931 book *Asanas*, Indra Devi in her 1953 *Forever Young, Forever Healthy*, and B.K.S. Iyengar, who developed his own branch of yoga and published *Light on Yoga* in 1965, all avoided the subject of injury. Guru Swami Gitananda, a veteran of world tours and developer of ashrams claimed, "Real yoga is as safe as mother's milk."[13]

My cousin Susan is the other half of my yoga-practicing family. My discussions with Susan, also tall and willowy, only twenty years older than Katie, were far more successful than with my niece. Susan agreed with Broad that, without proper caution, there is danger of injury in the practice of yoga. She pointed out that when she began sixteen years ago, yoga wasn't as popular as it is today. It was more of an oddity with the reputation (not entirely accurate) of being practiced by new-age types and ex-hippies. Classes were small, the teachers were experienced, and it was possible for teacher and student to know each other well. Susan has only ever had one teacher.

She also agreed with Black that the key to avoiding injury is to discuss any pre-existing physical problems with the teacher, and avoid any positions that are uncomfortable. Susan has never had an injury, and she never saw any of the students in her classes injured. There are some poses she just won't do—shoulder stands, for one. And if a position causes pain, she avoids it, a devotee of my philosophy: no pain is good. She came to yoga with a chronic groin problem dating from her middle school cheerleading days that caused her occasional pain. She and her teacher have worked on that problem over the years, and it has never been better controlled. The same goes for an issue with peripheral neuropathy affecting her feet and better management of her stress than she has ever been able to achieve with the help of professionals and pharmaceuticals. As she has traversed middle age, she feels yoga has kept her stronger and more fluid. Susan is an exception to my rule that everyone who exercises hurts themselves eventually. In my defense however, she did have that groin injury. And she is an excellent example of my philosophy that caution and moderation are a logical approach to improving safety.

Echoing the well-known advantages of yoga, Susan described her classmates, many of whom are also long-term followers of her teacher, as being in good health. Serious followers of the art develop a lifestyle that is healthy in general. They pay attention to good nutrition and stay active between yoga sessions. Susan hoola-hoops (I didn't know that was a verb). She also walks everywhere she can, often with her dog. She reiterated several times, as does Black, that the key to avoiding injury is to have a good teacher.

A concern of hers is that as yoga has become more popular the number of classes has exploded. Yoga has shown up in retirement communities and grade schools, and everywhere in-between. The number of teachers has climbed too, and their training and knowledge appear to be less robust than when the community was smaller and teacher education better controlled. A marginally trained teacher with a large class of students unknown to that teacher, all doing the same poses as the teacher who doesn't know the students' abilities or pre-existing injuries, is a recipe for disaster, according to all commentators. She has also heard of beginner students who are in an inappropriate class and feel intimidated into keeping up with the class and teacher when, in fact, they are unprepared to do so. An injury in that setting is likely to make one gun-shy about returning, much like my fractured rib did to me with Aikido. And an undiagnosed injury that one ignores for too long can lead to chronic pain and discomfort.

But people look to yoga to treat their aches and pains, not to make them worse. Susan also credits the type of yoga she practices, Iyengar Yoga, as helping to keep her injury-free. She describes it as a less aggressive form of yoga that uses straps, blankets, and blocks to help achieve and maintain poses. Other forms of yoga do the same. Susan's neighbor owns a Vinyasa Yoga studio and echoes her experience. She endeavors to know her students and advise them individually about how best to proceed with their practice and remain safe. Her pet peeve is the student who ignores her advice to avoid certain poses, is injured, and then blames her anyway! I feel her pain. As a physician, regardless of how carefully I explain the potential risks of surgery and possibility of failure, if there is less than a perfect outcome, I take the hit.

Broad references several medical journals in describing some of the more serious injuries seen in yoga practitioners, especially neurologic injuries. Reports began surfacing in the 1970s in *Neurology*, *The British Medical Journal*, and *The Journal of the American Medical Association*. An early case involved a young man who developed a foot drop—a condition in which the foot cannot be elevated at the ankle due to weakness of the muscles that run along the anterior lower leg and top of the foot. The result is a foot that stays in a "dropped" position and interferes with walking. The individual has difficulty with the toe catching when stepping forward or climbing a step and, as a result, tends to lift the foot higher to clear the sagging forefoot. As the foot comes down it creates a slapping sound. The high-stepped walk is known as a steppage gait. The most common cause is compression of a nerve root in the lumbar spine from a herniated disk or bone spur and is a component of the condition called sciatica. There are other causes, however.

This man, not long before he became weak, had started sitting in *vajrasana* for hours at a time. This is a common yoga seated position in which the lower leg is bent under the thighs and with the buttocks positioned over the soles of the feet. It puts the knee into 180 degrees of flexion, forced so by the entire weight of the upper body. The superficial peroneal nerve (SPN), a branch of the sciatic nerve, runs around the outer edge of the knee on its way to innervate the muscles that elevate the foot.

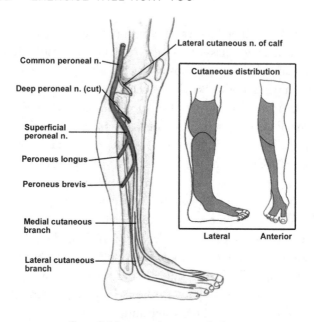

Superficial peroneal nerve at the knee.

The extreme position of the knee for hours at a time resulted in his foot drop by compressing the nerve and compromising its blood supply. The formal name of this condition is entrapment neuropathy, the most common example of which is carpal tunnel syndrome. Here the SPN is trapped under the tendons of the muscles that insert at the knee while simultaneously being stretched by the fully flexed knee. The foot drop, in this case, resolved once the cause was identified, and he gave up vajrasana. If the compression had gone on for long enough, the foot drop could have been permanent due to chronic ischemia (long-standing inadequate blood supply) of the nerve.

Cerebral ischemia leading to stroke is the most ominous example of the dangers inherent in yoga. The four arteries that supply the brain are two carotid arteries that run through the anterior neck and two smaller vertebral arteries that run in the posterior neck through bony channels lateral to the vertebral bodies that make up the cervical spine.

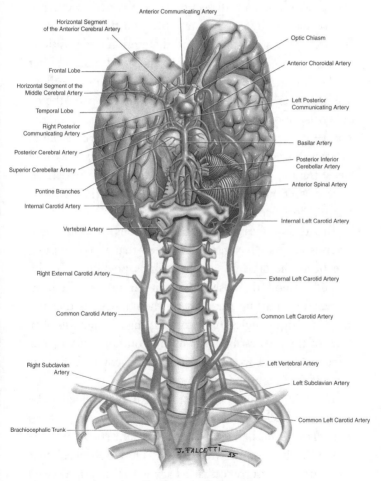

Cerebral vasculature.

Arterialdissection is a condition that develops when the inner wall of an artery tears and a channel develops between the inner and outer layers of the vessel wall, creating a false lumen that fills with blood that goes nowhere, but can collapse the true lumen of the artery and block its blood flow. The term dissection refers to the dissecting of the vessel wall by the fluid jet acting on the false lumen. The neck is highly mobile, and the motion and positions it can assume are transmitted to its blood vessels. That is the reason why dissections in younger people—those younger than the age group that has developed atherosclerosis, another cause of dissection, especially in the aorta—occur most commonly in the carotid and vertebral arteries. Yoga positions that hyperbend the neck can cause neck trauma, and neck trauma is frequently associated with dissection—though spontaneous dissection without trauma does occur.

Broad describes some of the positions that put these arteries at risk. "Iyengar emphasized that in cobra pose, the head should arch 'as far back as possible.'" In the shoulder stand, the pose my cousin will not do, the head is flexed by putting the chin on the chest such that the head is at right angles to the torso. Iyengar called this pose "one of the greatest boons conferred on humanity by our ancient sages." I wonder if he thinks it comes before or after ethical monotheism.

In 1972, neurophysiologist W. Ritchie Russell published an article in *The British Medical Journal* describing the relationship between yoga poses and stroke in otherwise healthy young individuals.[14] He emphasized that these are rare occurrences, and I agree. In thirty-nine years of practicing neurosurgery, I've seen my share of arterial dissections. I don't remember a single one caused by yoga. But there's yet another saying in medicine; something that happens only rarely, less than 1 percent of the time, happens 100 percent to the patient affected. The extreme postures assumed by the neck in certain yoga exercises can cause the very type of trauma to the carotid and vertebral arteries that is known to cause dissection.

Russell stressed the potential danger to the vertebral arteries that, by virtue of their forming the basilar artery, supply the brainstem and cerebellum. Strokes involving the brain stem can be devastating and, not uncommonly, fatal. All neurologic functions, those descending from the brain on the way to the body and those ascending from the body on the way to the brain, go through the brain stem, which is approximately the size of a thumb. Even a small area of damage to this most elegant area of the brain can cause widespread neurologic injury. The cerebellum, on the other hand, is considerably larger. It has significant input into normal and coordinated movement. Damage to it can produce ataxia (a muscle control problem), dizziness, vertigo, loss of coordination and postural instability. In humans, it is smaller than the cerebral cortex, that part of the brain associated with those characteristics that make us human—language, cognition, self-awareness and the ability to reason. In non-human animal species, which are more dependent on physical attributes for survival— speed, agility, strength, climbing and swimming—the cerebellum is considerably larger than the cerebral cortex. The brain stem and cerebellum are evolutionarily older parts of the brain than the cerebrum, and their asymmet-

ric importance in comparison to the cerebrum predates
the appearance of *Homo sapiens* and our progenitor homi-
nid species by hundreds of millions of years.

Not all dissections present with neurologic symptoms.
In my practice, the majority of these injuries do not cause
stroke and don't need intervention. Anticoagulation is
commonly used for several weeks, and the vessel eventually heals on its own. The most common and virtually
universal symptom of dissection is neck pain. A tear in the
wall of an artery is painful, and pressure over the involved
carotid or vertebral artery produces tenderness. The onset
of the symptoms is sudden. That history, in combination
with a recent neck injury in a young, active individual
with neck tenderness, is a classic presentation, easily recognized by a neurologist or neurosurgeon, but less likely
to be familiar to other physicians. Given the fact that
stroke is uncommon, and most yoga practitioners don't
consider their art a form of trauma, it's likely that there
are more dissections than are reported. Many are likely
unrecognized as dissections, and, in the event they are,
their relationship to yoga may go unnoticed. And even
without treatment with anticoagulation, they can heal
spontaneously.

Broad describes two cases from that rare, less than 1
percent of the time occurrence rate. The first was a patient
of Willibald Nagler of Cornell University, reported in
1973. A twenty-eight-year-old woman was in the upward
"wheel" pose that involves creating a reverse semicircular
arc with the body balanced on the hands and feet. She
briefly balanced her upper body on the vertex of her head
with her neck severely extended. She had the immedi-

ate onset of a severe headache and needed assistance in standing and walking. At the hospital she had symptoms of Wallenberg's Syndrome, a stroke involving the vertebral artery and, in particular, a branch called the posterior inferior cerebellar artery. In addition to ataxia, she had absence of sensation on her right side, weakness on her left side, a left gaze preference and a partial left Horner's syndrome ptosis (drooping eyelid), and meiosis (constriction of the pupil).

She was taken to surgery where her left cerebellar hemisphere was found to be infarcted (stroked) and much of the tissue dead. Two years later, she could walk—although with a wide-based gait—had poor coordination of her left arm, and residual abnormality of her left pupil and eyelid. Stroke symptoms that are still present two years after the event remain forever.

The second case comes from *The Archives of Neurology* in 1977, authored by Steven Hanus, M.D., and his colleagues. It is similar to the first case; a vertebral artery stroke in a twenty-five-year-old yoga participant. A veteran of daily yoga for a year and a half, he included extreme head rotation to the left and right in his routine. He would follow with the now-infamous shoulder stand with his head fully flexed. He developed the sudden onset of visual blurring, dysphagia (swallowing difficulty), and a left hemiparesis. Imaging revealed occlusion of the left vertebral artery. In this setting, traumatic arterial dissection is virtually always the cause. Two months after the stroke, he was still impaired, walking with a cane and with significant left hand weakness.

Arterial dissections as a result of yoga poses are vanishingly rare. That fact was used to criticize Broad as he made his way through the interview circuit. He references a 2009 Columbia University survey that asked yoga teachers, physicians, and physical therapists to describe the most serious yoga-related injuries they had seen. At the top of the list were lower back, shoulder, knee, and neck injuries, each numbering in the hundreds. Stroke was listed, but there were only four. Strokes from arterial injury are in fact more common in other sports, in particular in contact sports.

Paradoxically, yoga has been used to treat stroke victims during their recovery. A common sequela of stroke includes difficulty with balance and increased risk of falling. The fear of falling is a significant barrier in the rehabilitation of stroke victims, especially in the elderly. Physical therapists work to improve strength and balance in order to return patients to independent ambulation. In a study conducted at the Indianapolis Veterans Hospital and published in *Stroke* in July 2012, adding yoga to the rehab program of a subgroup of stroke patients provided several benefits in comparison to the non-yoga treated subgroups. There was statistically significant improvement in balance and reduction in fear of falling. Also noted was an improved quality of life and better independence with daily activities.[15]

Stroke was not the only yoga injury Broad discussed, and if his revelations save only a single yogi from assuming a pose that could cause a stroke, then he has fulfilled the Talmudic maxim that "to save a single soul is to save the entire world."[16] He quotes the Consumer Product Safety Commission that surveyed emergency room admissions due to yoga injuries. The number is still small but from 2000 to 2002 the number increased three and a half times, from thirteen to forty-six. The survey is done by sampling ERs rather than by collecting comprehensive reporting data. The total number is therefore understated. The trend of the increase, however, is statistically accurate. Additionally, only a small fraction of yoga injuries are assumed to necessitate an ER visit, and, in the eleven years since this survey, the number of yoga participants has continued to increase.

Broad ends his article by taking us back to Glenn Black, whom he introduced in his opening sentence. Black ultimately needed back surgery for spinal stenosis, undergoing a lumbar laminectomy and fusion. He blames his many decades of yoga for causing the problem. He's only partially correct. Spinal stenosis is an almost universal component of aging and is present to some degree in nearly 100 percent of people over sixty. It's not always symptomatic, and most of us never require surgery. But an active lifestyle can definitely contribute to its development. It is after all, a 'wear-and-tear' phenomenon. If you wear more, you will tear more, yoga included.

The potential hazards of yoga have not been ignored, even by those who were annoyed with Broad's *Times* article. Over the past decade, *Yoga Journal* has increased their coverage of this issue. Its editor and increasing numbers of instructors have gone public with their own injuries and how they've altered their teaching styles to deal with those of their students. One prominent Iyengar instructor and frequent contributor to *Yoga Journal* has stressed the dangers of extreme bending of the neck and recommended against doing our old friend the shoulder stand without a modification that allows for a lesser degree of neck angulation.

The medical editor of the journal highlighted the dangers of doing headstands and suggested they should not be done in general yoga classes. His own use of the pose led to thoracic outlet syndrome, another of the entrapment neuropathies, in which the nerves of the brachial plexus that run behind the clavicle are compressed. He developed numbness and tingling in the arm and hand. Untreated it can cause arm and hand weakness. A physician, he recognized the problem and its relationship to the headstands and stopped doing them. His symptoms cleared in time. He also cautioned that headstands can accelerate the development of degenerative arthritis of the cervical spine and cause eye damage secondary to the increase in ocular pressure from inversion. Individuals with glaucoma are at particular risk when using any kind of inversion therapy or pose. Due to the already increased ocular pressure in glaucoma, further increasing it by inverting oneself carries a real risk of producing sudden, and permanent, blindness. This is especially so if glaucoma is undiagnosed and the individual is not being treated. Fortunately, glaucoma is not common. It affects approximately 0.5 percent of the adult population under fifty. In those over eighty, its incidence is 10 percent.

Yoga. Blinding pain. I didn't see that one coming.

Chapter 3

COMPETITIVE, CONTACT EXERCISE: BOXING, FOOTBALL, AND HOCKEY

BOXING

"Martial": word connoting the military, and war. These are the sports that involve fighting. I'm not sure which is the oldest, but wrestling was known among the Greeks and was included in the original Olympic Games. The self-defense arts, such as Judo and Karate, most having originated in Asia, are probably at least as old. But the one that stands out from all the rest, especially for me, is boxing.

It too dates back to at least the Greeks, who thought it was a sport of their gods. Homer references boxing in the *Iliad*. Written in the eighth century BCE, it is the story of the Trojan War, which dates to the thirteenth century

BCE. Like the gladiator battles also popular in ancient Rome, boxing became at times a fight to the death. A form of the modern boxing glove of today made its appearance at that time. Competitors would protect their hands by wrapping them with leather straps, which at times would have metal added to them to make the fight that much more lethal.

After the fall of Rome, little was heard about boxing until eighteenth century England when it was unregulated and covered by no organized rule system. The fights consisted of unprotected bare fists in matches that had no time constraints. It was little more than a planned two-man street fight.

In 1866 the Marquess of Queensberry proposed rules that became incorporated into the sport and are named for him. They included the mandatory use of gloves and a three-minute time limit on each of a pre-set number of rounds. In the 160 years since, the popularity of the sport has grown, and the rules are now regulated by several professional organizations. Champions of the sport have become among the world's most recognizable athletes and, in the modern era, none more so than Muhammad Ali.[1]

As a neurosurgeon, I have taken care of more than a thousand head-injured patients. I have seen every kind, from the minor to the fatal, caused by all manner of trauma, both accidental and intentional. I've seen closed head injuries and open ones; blunt force trauma and penetrating injuries; simple bumps caused by falls from standing height; and crushing injuries from high-speed vehicular accidents. I've seen injuries that the best make-up artist in Hollywood can't come close to.

What then am I, a neurosurgeon, supposed to think of a sport, the object of which is to create in your opponent a head injury of sufficient severity so as to render him unconscious? The knockout is the goal of the boxer, at least at the professional level. The brutality and viciousness of boxing evoke its ancient origins and those gladiators of Rome.

There is certainly the blood. Facial lacerations are a universal part of the sport. Subcutaneous bleeding that swell eyes shut are commonplace. There's even a maneuver known as cutting, in which the tense, swollen eyelid is intentionally incised to allow the blood to drain, reducing the pressure and reopening the eye.

The force that is applied to the head is astronomical. As training methods improved and performance-enhancing drugs such as steroids came into common usage, the strength and quickness of professional boxers improved as well. We've all seen the slow-motion movie sequences of boxing matches where close-up views show us the fist slamming into the face, the nose and lips being grotesquely disfigured as the head snaps around, sweat and blood flying into the crowd. In a "kill shot" you can see awareness disappear from the eyes as the boxer falls unprotected and slams his head again on the ring floor. This is not a sport. This is a vestige of some dark, brutal era when people were forced to fight to the death, against each other or some wild animal, while spectators cheered and hooted from the safety of the amphitheater.

It should be banned. I am not the first to suggest that. Among others during the modern era of boxing, the *Journal of the American Medical Association,* made the same recommendation in 1983.[2]

I touched on concussions earlier. They have been getting a great deal of attention in recent years, and research has shown them to be far more pernicious an injury than was once thought. A classic concussion is defined as a head injury producing immediate loss of consciousness, lasting usually seconds to minutes. Upon awakening, the individual is usually disoriented, often amnestic about the injury, and recovers over the subsequent hours or days. These are the injuries the coach would tell us to "walk off," as if pacing up and down the sideline would make the effects of the injury wear off more quickly in the hope of returning the player to the game, especially if he or she was a star performer. That is a dangerous thing to do.

Not all concussions, however, require the loss of consciousness to be classified as such. We now know that any head injury that causes any type of change in mental status is technically a concussion. This includes the "bell ringers," which stun a player and may make him or her woozy, unsteady, confused, and may cause a blank stare, slurred speech, or double vision. The technical term for this group of head injuries is mild Traumatic Brain Injury, or TBI.

TBI is a spectrum of injury that spans the range from very mild, as are concussions, to the catastrophic and fatal. Pathophysiology is the science of injury—the damage to or disease of an organism or organ system that causes it to dysfunction. The abnormality can exist on the macroscopic level, such as an anatomic change seen with, for example, a fractured leg; the microscopic level, such as a bacterial infection that invades cellular structures; or the biochemical level that exists in the submicroscopic world of proteins, DNA, and the chemical interactions that govern all life. In virtually all disease states, all three levels co-exist.

A brain injury, at its most basic, is any process that prevents normal neuronal transmission. The brain is a vastly complex collection of billions of nerves, known as neurons. Each neuron consists of a nerve cell body from which two types of structures project.

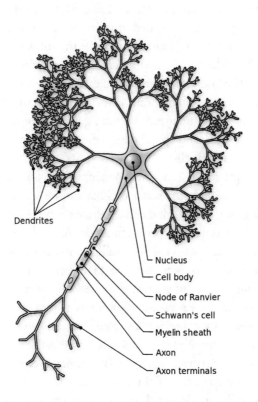

Dendrites

Nucleus

Cell body

Node of Ranvier

Schwann's cell

Myelin sheath

Axon

Axon terminals

Nerve cell.

Dendrites are the thinner and shorter of the two, and there can be multiple dendrites from each cell body. They traverse between cell bodies and provide intercommunication between neurons. The axon is the longer and thicker of the projections. The cell body is superficial in the brain, located in the gyrus, the multiply infolded structures that give the brain its convoluted surface appearance. The color of the brain's surface is gray and is called the gray matter.

The axon leaves the cell and becomes coated with an insulating substance called myelin, which functions to facilitate neuronal transmission of the nerve impulse. Myelin is white and gives its color to the internal structures of the brain known as white matter. The axons travel into the depths of the brain carrying the nerve impulses to the deeper structures, the basal ganglia, the thalamus, the brain stem, and spinal cord, where they connect with still other nerve cells.

This progression of interconnecting nerves continues until the end organ is reached. That can be a muscle that causes movement, a gland that releases a hormone, or an organ that has its own specific function. Along the way, each neuron is interconnected with millions of others by way of the dendritic processes, creating the original internet and consisting of an estimated one hundred trillion connections. The network serves as an unknowably complex system of billions of modifying inputs from one nerve to another, resulting in actions as mundanely reflexive as the blink of an eye, and as mystifyingly elegant as a human thought.

It is the anatomy of the brain that creates its susceptibility to injury. When I give lectures on head injury to medical students and residents, I remind them of the college requirements for admission to medical school, one of which is at least one course in physics. At times, the need for having had to suffer through physics, which is largely applied calculus, is obscure. Although there were those among us pre-medical undergraduates who found this science elegant, its applicability in the day-to-day practice of medicine can be difficult to discern.

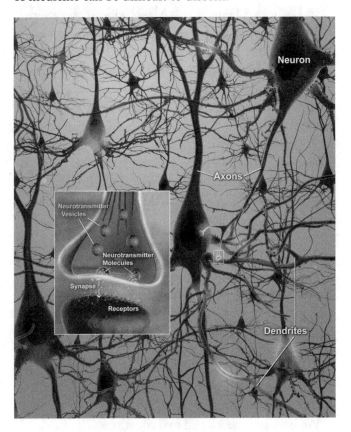

Neuronal interconnections.

Except in the treatment of TBI, which neurosurgeons see all the time. I remind my students of Isaac Newton's second law of motion, an equation they learned in Physics 101:

$$F=MA$$

It tells us that Force equals Mass times Acceleration. It is a versatile equation. It helped put astronauts into space, in part explains Johannes Kepler's observations of planetary motion, and explains why the human brain poorly tolerates sudden changes in its state of motion.

An injury is created by an object striking the head at rest, or a head in motion striking an object that causes a sudden alteration in that motion—not uncommonly, an instantaneous complete stop. Because the nerve's anatomy changes as it transforms from the cell body in the gray matter (gm) to the axon in the white matter (wm), its mass changes also. Therefore,

$$M(gm) \text{ does not equal } M(wm).$$

Stay with me. This is after all, physics.

The force applied to the head by the injuring object, however, is applied equally to both the gray matter and the white matter, and therefore,

$$F(gm) = F(wm).$$

We have now developed two equations,

$$F(gm) = M(gm) \times A(gm)$$
$$\text{and}$$
$$F(wm) = M(wm) \times A(wm).$$

Because the effect of the injuring force is equal to both parts of the neuron, and the left sides of the equations are in equality, then the right sides of the equations must also be equal, and

$$M(gm) \times A(gm) = M(wm) \times A(wm).$$

But, as we know, the masses are not equal. So the accelerations cannot be equal, and therefore

$$A(gm) \text{ does not equal } A(wm).$$

In head injury, a stationary brain suddenly moved by a striking object accelerates. A moving brain suddenly stopped negatively accelerates, that is, it decelerates. The above reasoning tells us that the portion of the neuron in the gray matter accelerates or decelerates at a different rate than the portion of the neuron in the white matter.

Imagine a soft spaghetti noodle, stretched tightly and moving through space. If it was to come to a sudden stop, and the top and bottom halves of the noodle stopped at different rates, the noodle would bend. If the force were great enough, the noodle would tear.

The neuron reacts similarly. This differential motion sustained by different parts of the same neuron as a result of the force of the injury causes damage to the nerve at the point where it traverses the transition zone from gray to white matter, called the gray-white junction.

If the injury is mild, the nerve function is temporarily disrupted. This is an injury at the biochemical level. Neuronal transmission is an electrical event created by the movement of sodium, potassium, and calcium ions passing back and forth across the cell membrane of the neuron. The injury disrupts this process, and the neuron ceases to function. If enough neurons are affected, there are neurologic changes, the most dramatic being a classic concussion, the sudden loss of consciousness I described above, that is caused by the widespread cessation of neuronal function. Common examples of this type of injury are the numbness or tingling that occur when your legs are crossed for too long and your foot "falls asleep." Another is the electrical shock–like sensation and subsequent tingling in the hand when you hit your elbow and traumatize the ulnar nerve, popularly referred to as the "crazy bone."

These are temporary nerve injuries. The neuron is injured but still intact, as are all the support structures of the nerve, including the myelin sheath, and the nerve will recover, often quickly, as in the above examples. The technical name for this nerve injury is neurapraxia. As recovery occurs, the symptoms resolve; the injured athlete awakens, the asleep foot stops tingling. In the case of concussion, symptoms other than unconsciousness can persist for longer periods of time. I will discuss those later.

If the injury is more severe, there can be actual disruption of the axon within its encasing structures, but the latter remain intact. The axon will degenerate beyond the point of injury, a process called Wallerian Degeneration, but because all the nerve sheaths are intact, the nerve can regenerate over time by growing back along those preserved sheaths. The neurologic consequences are worse and longer-lasting. Recovery can occur as the neurons regenerate, but there are often errors in this process, and scarring at the site of the axonal damage can prevent complete healing. As a result, residual symptoms and neurologic deficits are common. It can take a year or more for the recovery to reach its end point. The technical name in this injury is axonotmesis.

In the worst-case scenario, the injuring force is great enough to cause complete disruption of the entire neuronal structure: the axon, the support structures, and the myelin sheath. In this setting the neurons are commonly severed. These are devastating injuries from which recovery is not possible. The victim is immediately rendered unconscious and enters a state of deep coma. There are often concomitant injuries to other parts of the body, and there is a high fatality rate in this population. Automobile and motorcycle accidents are frequent mechanisms of these injuries. With time the site of the injury to the nerve scars over, and the attempt by the nerve to regenerate is thwarted by its inability to traverse the scar and find the tubular sheath it needs to grow into, for it too is no longer in continuity. This is called neurotmesis.

The latter two types of TBI are referred to as diffuse axonal injury, DAI.

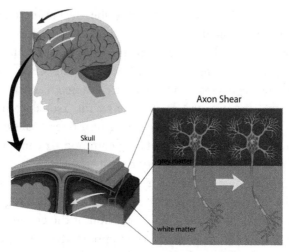

Illustration of diffuse axonal injury (DAI).

These are injuries on all three levels I described—anatomic, cellular, and biochemical. The injuries to the neurons can be seen on MRI or CT scans of the brain and represent small hemorrhages at the grey-white junction.

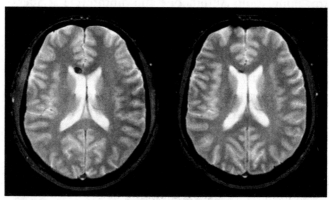

MRI of DAI (small black ovals) at three days (*left*) and four months (*right*).

They are called shear injuries, the name derived from the description of what has occurred to the neurons as a result of the differential deceleration. If the patient survives, disability is common. In the most severely injured group, those with neurotmesis, survivors are left in a persistent vegetative state. This is a condition of total disability. The patient appears awake, but is fully disconnected from the environment. He or she can't speak, follows no commands, and gives no indication that he or she is aware of anyone or anything. He or she is fed through a tube inserted directly into the stomach or small intestine. There is usually a tracheotomy to allow suctioning and clearing of the airway. The patient requires around-the-clock care and will for the remainder of his life.

There is another peculiarity of the anatomy of the brain that needs explaining to fully understand the pathophysiology of TBI. The brain is a soft organ encased in a rigid inelastic container, the skull. Within the confines of the skull, the brain floats in a liquid medium called CSF or cerebrospinal fluid. CSF is produced in the ventricular system, a series of four cavities in the center of the brain. This fluid travels through the ventricles and exits from them at the base of the brain through three openings called foramina. The CSF then circulates over the surface of the brain and spinal cord under a gossamer structure called the arachnoid membrane, creating a CSF-filled space, the subarachnoid space. It is this fluid that is sampled during a lumbar puncture, better known as a spinal tap, done to diagnose nervous system diseases such as meningitis, among others.

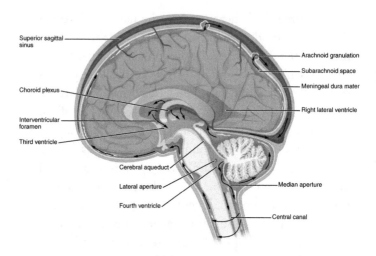

Superior sagittal sinus

Arachnoid granulation

Subarachnoid space

Meningeal dura mater

Choroid plexus

Right lateral ventricle

Interventricular foramen

Third ventricle

Cerebral aqueduct

Lateral aperture

Median aperture

Fourth ventricle

Central canal

CSF circulation

In general the skull and brain move as a unit; whatever motion is applied to the skull is equally applied to the brain, similar to what I explained in the discussion above concerning force applied to the brain. In the case of a severe sudden motion, or force, the brain can shake within the skull. With my students, I use the image of a bowl of Jell-O to illustrate. Imagine holding that bowl and shaking it. The Jell-O will shake too, but when you stop the motion of the bowl, the Jell-O continues to shake a few more times, bouncing back-and-forth off the inside walls of the container.

The brain will do the same thing if the head comes to a sudden stop. In addition to the effect on the axons at the grey-white junction as I've explained, the brain, floating in the sea of CSF, will continue to shake and impact against the inner surface of the skull. It will strike first against the side of the skull toward which the head is traveling and then ricochet in the opposite direction striking the surface of the skull on the direct opposite side of the head. For example, if you are running downfield with the football when you are met head-on by a defender who inadvertently hits your head with his, your head will come to a sudden stop. Your brain will continue to travel forward striking the inner surface of your frontal bone, then bounce back in the opposite direction striking the inner surface of the occipital bone, or the back of the head.

This injury has its own name, a coup-contrecoup injury. The coup injury is the first strike going forward. The contrecoup injury is the second strike on the bounce back.

This is the most common mechanism of injury causing a concussion. If the injury force is more severe than usual, an actual contusion of the brain can result. This is bruising on the surface of the brain that can be seen on a CT scan as an area of bleeding (unlike concussion, which is associated with a negative CT scan). If there is a coup-contrecoup contusion, there will be two visible areas of bleeding, 180 degrees apart, or opposite each other in the brain. If the bleeding is substantial, it can break through the brain surface and collect between the brain and the skull. Known as a subdural hemorrhage, if large enough, it can be fatal and requires emergency surgery to remove the clot. It is uncommon in athletic competition.

In sport, the mildest of these injuries is the most common, reminding one of the axiom of logic that tells us the most common things happen most commonly. In medicine we tell our students that when they hear hoof-beats, don't think of zebras. When trying to diagnose a complex of symptoms, think of the common causes (horses), not the uncommon ones (zebras). As a corollary of this reasoning, I see a lot of concussions, especially in the warm weather months when outdoor activities abound.

Contusions are less common, and DAI is rare, but not unheard of. I started this discussion with a description of mild TBI, a concussion. What follows here is what follows the concussion once the initial event passes. Although some concussions clear completely within hours of the injury, most last for a few days, and it is not uncommon for them to leave the individual symptomatic for weeks or months. They do however resolve eventually. But for the patient with this problem, eventually can seem endless.

The constellation of symptoms that follow a mild TBI is called post concussion syndrome (PCS). It includes a long list of possible complaints that can occur together or in isolation. Headache is the hallmark of the syndrome and affects virtually all concussed individuals. Dizziness, visual disturbance, unsteadiness, ear ringing, personality changes, memory loss, difficulty concentrating, shortened attention span, deterioration in school performance, insomnia, and fatigue, are some of the many problems I have seen in patients with TBI. There is very recent information that provides an enlarging picture of just how insidious and damaging the accumulated effects of repetitive mild TBI can be. An expanding body of knowledge suggests that severe, possibly debilitating changes in brain anatomy can occur with what on the surface appear to be insignificant injuries.

PCS can last, rarely, a few hours; more commonly days or weeks. A minority will last several months, and, also rarely, up to a year. There are no curative treatments for PCS, but its symptoms can be addressed. Pain can be medicated, and for persistent cognitive changes there is psychological counseling. A branch of physical therapy known as vestibular therapy is helpful in dealing with symptoms of unsteadiness, gait and balance issues, and visual disturbances. Time is the real healer. This is what is known as a self-limited disease, one that disappears on its own. Much like the common cold that lasts a week if you do nothing but disappears in seven days if you treat it, PCS will resolve with time. Its symptoms can be debilitating at worst and are always annoying. When all the symptoms have disappeared, one is considered recovered.

In young children with concussion, there is information that complete cognitive rest is the best treatment. This involves removing all stimulation from the child. No schoolwork, reading, watching TV, video games, computer use, playing with friends. None. Nothing. As a parent of three children who were young at one point, I can't think of anything more difficult to pull off than that. I'm not yet convinced the research supports that drastic a treatment protocol, and intuitively it seems that the frustration of a child cut off from everything would be counterproductive. I do instruct my patients, or their parents, to get as much sleep and other forms of rest as possible, avoid stressors of any kind, halt work or school and recreation, and relax. But activity that is easily tolerated, and at times necessary, is reasonable. With time, more activity will be tolerable. I rely on my philosophy that if it doesn't hurt, it's OK. An activity that doesn't cause or worsen symptoms is permitted. The individual can be trusted, in most cases, to do the right thing with a little guidance. That prescription has worked for me for thirty years. I'll continue to follow it until irrefutable evidence suggests otherwise.

Once all the symptoms have resolved, it is then, and only then, that you can return to the activity that caused the injury. Most of these sports are those where contact is a part of the game. Boxing is only the most egregious of them. Football, lacrosse, ice hockey, basketball, soccer, diving, riding (anything—animal or vehicle), are just some of the more common ones. If there is any chance that additional head contact might occur, returning to the sport while symptoms persist is dangerous in the extreme.

Julian Bailes—chairman of the Department of Neurosurgery at the West Virginia University School of Medicine, in Morgantown, West Virginia until 2011—has been studying mild TBI for several decades. Using his proximity to Pittsburgh, Pennsylvania, he has recruited the members of the football teams at both the University of Pittsburgh, a NCAA Division I team, and the Pittsburgh Steelers of the NFL as study subjects. He is currently at North Shore University in Evanston, Illinois, and the University of Chicago.

Choosing these athletes to follow after TBI has distinct advantages. They are all highly motivated individuals committed to their sport. They want to return to playing at the earliest possible time. In any scientific study, the results are most reliable when the factors that can skew results are eliminated. In studying concussion, not being absolutely sure of when PCS symptoms have resolved is an example of one of those factors. If the injured individual doesn't want to return to their pre-injury job, or has litigation pending from the injury, the actual time it takes for the symptoms of TBI to clear may be exaggerated. Conversely, an athlete who is chomping at the bit to get back in the game won't malinger. The problem is just the opposite. They might downplay, or deny altogether, persistent symptoms. There are tests that can help determine if the injury has resolved, but they are not foolproof. Remember, the symptoms of PCS are largely subjective, and in most cases can't be measured. If someone tells me they still have a headache or are dizzy after an injury, or if they have those symptoms and tell me they don't, there is no objective test to disprove the claim.

Bailes and his team at the Brain Injury Research Institute at WVU did careful neurological and psychological evaluations of the team members at the start and at the end of the season. He did additional testing of injured players. He also used MRI and PET scanning to follow the injuries.

In 2008, testifying before Congress, he revealed some of the findings of his research. Using data from retired NFL players, he found a surprisingly high incidence of cognitive problems. Retired players not only had a higher incidence of mild cognitive impairment (MCI) than the general, age-matched population, but the only risk factor discovered was that they'd had three or more concussions during their professional career. In those cases, the chance of having MCI was five times higher. It is recognized that in this setting, the majority of these athletes will develop Alzheimer's disease within ten years.[3]

A second study, looking at psychological changes, found an 11 percent incidence of depression in the retirees. Again, this is three times the expected incidence for the general population. The same three-concussion risk factor was found.[4]

A disturbing finding that has come out of increasing attention to mild TBI is the phenomenon of second injury, or second impact syndrome. It is now clear that a concussion significantly increases the likelihood that a subsequent concussion will be more severe, even if the mechanism of the injury is similar to the previous one. The brain is primed, in some as yet unknown way, to be more easily damaged. The period of unconsciousness or disorientation is often longer. The post-concussion symptoms are more severe and last longer, and the chance of permanent brain damage is higher.

Concussions have ended the careers of several well-known athletes, and probably should have ended many others. Steve Young, the Hall of Fame quarterback for the San Francisco 49ers, played fourteen seasons between 1985–99. He had seven concussions that were documented in his NFL career and, likely, several others. He retired because of them, although he was contemplating returning for a fifteenth season at the time.

Eric Lindros of the NHL had a similar end to his career. At six-feet-four-inches and 240 pounds, he was the number one player taken in the 1991 NHL draft. He had size, speed, and strength, and was expected to be a hockey superstar. When he was healthy, his play dominated the league. In 1995 he won the Hart Trophy given to the sport's most valuable player. Unfortunately, his career was plagued by a variety of injuries. He had eight concussions in the era when this injury was taken far less seriously than it is today. While in Philadelphia playing for the Flyers, there was a very public controversy about the handling of his injuries, and Lindros feuded with both the Flyer management and team doctors about his care. In 2007, after fifteen seasons, he too retired.

Boxing is replete with examples of the lasting effects of repetitive head injury. For as long as there have been boxers, participants in the sport have been aware that long years in the ring can lead to being "punch drunk," a state of permanent brain damage with several names, the most colorful of which is dementia pugilistica (DP). DP is one of several types of brain injury that fall into the category of chronic traumatic encephalopathy (CTE), the damage that accrues slowly but steadily over time from repetitive blows to the head. Some come from those ferocious strikes that cause the unconsciousness of the knockout. But each punch, every jab, all the hits that snap the head, leave their imprint on the brain. Over time, the trillions of neuronal connections that create the network that constitutes normal brain function begin to die off.

The functional changes that result are those of dementia. Alzheimer's disease, a degenerative brain disease that also causes dementia, is common enough in the US that most of us know someone with this devastating, life ending condition. The dementia of the boxer is the same. Over time, clarity of thought fades. Confusion regarding even the simplest of tasks builds. Short-term memory disappears quickly, as does the ability to process new memories. Long-term memories take longer to disappear, but with time, even the people who are closest to the patient become strangers, having to reintroduce themselves with each meeting.

Independence slips away. Early on one can live at home with supervision. Eventually, something eludes the eyes of the family, and there's a near or actual miss. A stove is left on, starting a fire, or more commonly, the individual wanders away from the house, becoming lost, fearful, and defenseless. Some don't make it home. Others need to be put in a nursing facility where there is twenty-four hour observation. As mental capacity continues to deteriorate, ambulation becomes impossible, leading to life in a wheelchair. Once the ability to sit upright is gone, life speeds toward its end, the sufferer curled up in a bed, unaware, unknowing and alone except for the family at his side, who are strangers to him.

Several well-known boxers are reputed to have suffered from DP. Among them are Floyd Patterson, Jerry Quarry, Mike Quarry, Sugar Ray Robinson, and Meldrick Taylor.[5] Some of these athletes had their careers cut short. Others retired voluntarily only to have the symptoms develop later, no less life-altering.

Arguably, the best-known boxer to suffer from boxing-related brain damage is Muhammad Ali. Pugilistic Parkinson's Disease is another of the chronic traumatic encephalopathies and is well known to have afflicted the former champ because of the very public life he has maintained despite the debility of his disease. Parkinson's disease (PD) is a degenerative process that affects an area deep in the center of the brain known as the substantia nigra. The neurons of this area of the brain normally produce a neurotransmitter called dopamine. As the nerve cells degenerate, likely in the case of Ali as a result of repeated blows to his head, too little dopamine is available for normal nerve functioning, and symptoms appear.

PD is the most common of a group of neurologic disorders known as movement disorders. The earliest symptoms usually involve muscle function. Tremors, muscle rigidity, difficulty with gait and posture, and slow movement known as bradykinesia, are all common and debilitating. Medications that replenish dopamine, such as Sinemet, can make life significantly better, but they have their own disturbing side effects and can lose effectiveness with time. Deep brain stimulation, the introduction of electrodes into the thalamus of the brain connected to an implanted electrical generator, can have a dramatic impact on intractable tremors and has had a major impact on the treatment of this class of diseases.

In the late stages of PD, dementia is also common, attesting to the overlapping effects of the brain trauma of repetitive concussions. All the dementing diseases have a similar clinical course. The pace of decline varies from patient to patient, but the direction is always the same, downhill. Whether it is caused by degeneration of unknown cause, or by multiple concussive blows to the head, the result is the same. And it is never good.

Boxing at the non-professional level tries to reduce the danger inherent in the sport. Protective headgear and body pads are part of this level of boxing. Coaching is as concerned with safety as with fighting technique, all of which does lessen the potential damage. But boxing is a lot like smoking cigarettes. There is no way to smoke a cigarette safely. It is bad for you in all its manifestations. A concussion with head protection in place is still a concussion. It's not really the glove striking the head that does the damage. It is the brain, rocking back-and-forth and slamming against the inside of the skull as a result of the impact to the head, that does the damage. The result is the same.

I reiterate: boxing should be banned.

FOOTBALL

The concern about football is not a recent one. In 1905, there were nineteen documented deaths in college football. After a highly publicized beating taken by a player in the Penn-Swarthmore game in that year, President Theodore Roosevelt convened a meeting of the presidents of Princeton, Harvard and Yale to discuss the dangers of the game. At the time, there was little if any regulation of football, and the rules were lax in terms of protecting the players. Shailer Mathews, then the dean of the University of Chicago Divinity School, described football as follows: "From the President of the United States to the humblest member of a school and college faculty there arises a general protest against this boy-killing, man-mutilating, money making, education prostituting, gladiatorial sport."[6] Roosevelt, however, was a strong proponent of athletics and physical fitness; thus, despite calls to ban the game, he instead moved the colleges to establish better oversight. Penn was the first university to adopt rule changes, and several colleges in New York followed suit. In 1906, the Intercollegiate Athletics Association of the United States was formed to institutionalize the new rules. In 1910, this organization became the NCAA.[7]

A century later, in April 2010, twenty-one-year-old Owen Thomas, the captain of the University of Pennsylvania football team, committed suicide. An autopsy of his brain revealed chronic traumatic encephalopathy (CTE), which I discussed above in relation to boxing.

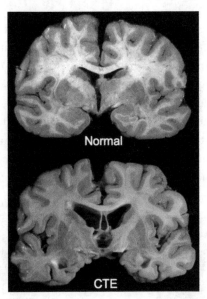

Micrographs of normal brain and CTE brain.

The disturbing fact in Thomas's case is that he never had a severe *single* injury. His mother stated that she believed her son had never suffered a single concussion. But his brain revealed the same changes seen in more than twenty deceased NFL players.[8]

In the absence of obvious head injuries, this finding suggests that the minor but frequent jolts that the head suffers even at the most junior stages of football competition can be additive. Quoting Thomas's mother again: "This is a person getting many little hits, starting at a young age. Football linebackers may get a thousand little hits. Now we're thinking these are like teaspoons. A thousand teaspoons of water could be the same as a big jug. It's possible."[9]

No one has suggested that the CTE was the direct cause, or causal in any way, of Thomas's taking his life. CTE is, however, associated with depression and impulse control issues. Two former NFL players who also committed suicide had CTE found at autopsy, including Junior Seau, an All-Pro linebacker who played twenty seasons in the league. The link for now is speculative. But this information has the attention of head injury researchers, and more will certainly be heard about this in the future.

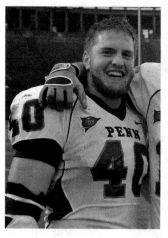 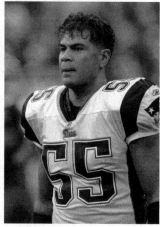

CTE suicides Owen Thomas (*left*) and Junior Seau (*right*).

The scientific evidence for a relationship between pathologic changes in the brain and repetitive concussions is just beginning to emerge. In April 2013, McCrory and associates, writing in *The British Journal of Sports Medicine,* published a study looking at that issue. The paper is a comprehensive review of the available evidence for CTE in retired professional athletes.[10]

For the purposes of their research, which was a large-scale review of existing literature, they classified concussion into four subsets based largely on descriptive criteria:

- Prolonged post concussive symptoms, which resolve completely.
- Persistent post concussion symptoms lasting longer than three months, with eventual full recovery. Structural neuroimaging is normal.
- Permanent PCS- representing 10 to 20 percent of the persistent PCS group. Functional and psychological testing may be abnormal but structural imaging is typically normal.
- CTE, where neurologic dysfunction exists and on postmortem examination neuropathologic changes are found to be present in the brain. Neuroimaging during life is often abnormal.

The authors add a note on the last group—there are individuals showing signs of CTE in life without pathologic changes found in the brain at autopsy. An additional caveat noted in this study is the effect on accurate diagnosis of these conditions during life caused by co-existing neurobehavioral health issues (known as co-morbidities) such as depression, personality disorders, anxiety, attention disorders, and the like.

Because there is little understanding of the physiologic changes that occur in the brain as a result of concussion, it is unclear where in the brain the symptoms of PCS are localized. There is no injury site that can be pinpointed as the cause of headache, fatigue, diminished concentration, sleep disturbance, and the many other symptoms that comprise PCS.[11] It is therefore not entirely clear if the above four-category description is a continuum of increasing severity of a single injury called mild traumatic brain injury, or whether these are distinct injury types that are independent entities. The prevailing opinion is that they are the former.

Diffusion tensor imaging (DTI) is a type of magnetic resonance imaging (MRI) that is particularly sensitive to alterations in the structure of the white matter of the frontal lobes. In January 2013, *Pediatric Neurology* published a paper by Virji-Babul and others from the University of Calgary. They looked at DTI changes in the white matter of adolescents with a sports related concussion occurring within two months of imaging. Importantly, they had a control group of age-matched subjects without a history of concussion.[12] Each individual underwent both a standard MRI scan to look at the structural anatomy of the brain, then each had two DTI scans. Physicians blinded to the characteristics of the participants read the scans. Additionally, each subject was assessed with the Sports Concussion Assessment Tool 2, a clinical examination incorporating a variety of postconcussion symptoms, physical signs, and coordination. A lower score is associated with injury.

Although the numbers were small, twelve test subjects and ten controls, the results were revealing and reached statistical significance. The authors observed clear differences in the white matter of the concussed athletes compared to their healthy control counterparts. There was widespread, bilateral change in the injured individuals. In addition, the Sports Concussion Assessment Tool 2 was a sensitive predictor of the changes on DTI. A score indicative of injury was associated with DTI changes, and the lower the score, the greater the abnormal findings on the scans.[13]

Given that the white matter is the part of the brain through which travel the myelinated nerve axons (the myelin imparting the white color to this part of the brain), these findings make intuitive sense. The widely accepted theory of the mechanism of concussion is that the injury creates stretching of the axons. That stretching results in their functioning improperly, producing the symptoms of concussion.

This study is one of the first to show a definitive link between mild TBI and the alteration of brain anatomy. There is no autopsy data to confirm this link because concussion victims do not die. And there remains a wide gap between the DTI data and the pathologic findings in the brains of athletes who have suffered repetitive mild TBI and have developed the life-altering symptoms of CTE later in life. We know what their brains look like because they do die. There is the suggestion of a link, however. The qualitative descriptions of the appearance of CTE brains, which include atrophy of the frontal and temporal lobes, match the sites where DTI imaging changes were found in the Calgary study.

In 1928, Dr. Harrison Martland, who coined the term "punch drunk," described what has become known as classic CTE, the symptom complex associated with professional boxers.[14] Typical symptoms include difficulty with speech, movement, and memory. A subset without memory involvement looks very much like Parkinson's Disease, named Pugilistic Parkinson's and, as I mentioned before, is most famously evident in Mohammed Ali. The neuropathologic changes found in these brains are well known and include cellular loss, scarring, and neuro-fibrillary tangles, a peculiar finding associated with brain injury.[15]

As information about the problems of retired NFL and NHL athletes became more available, a slightly different clinical syndrome has emerged. Although the symptoms of classic CTE can be present, neuropsychiatric and behavioral symptoms tend to show up earlier. Among them: depression, paranoia, agitation, social withdrawal and aggression.[16, 17, 18] Not associated with classic CTE, these symptoms progress in varying degrees to dementia. McCrory calls this modern CTE in his paper.[19] There are similarities found in the brains of both groups of CTE patients. The frontotemporal atrophy mentioned above is more characteristic of modern CTE.

The findings described in boxers' brains do show up in cases of modern CTE. But there is a specific finding in the brains of the modern form of the disease not found in the classic form. McKee and coworkers found an accumulation of tau-immunoreactive astrocytes, brain cells that contain the abnormal protein tau, that express themselves as filamentous tau lesions in the modern CTE brain. These filaments do not belong there.[20] As I will discuss later, there is some evidence to suggest that this same abnormal tau protein can show up in the spinal cords of patients with amyotrophic lateral sclerosis, a degenerative disease of the spinal cord, suggesting to some a link between repetitive concussions and ALS.[21]

The conclusions that can be reached from this information must be drawn with caution. There is still no conclusive evidence that CTE is a single entity, or that it comes solely from trauma. The constellation of symptoms overlap with other diseases that could be co-present in patients diagnosed with CTE, and that is especially true for the behavioral symptoms, the cause of which in many cases is poorly understood. But the trends certainly seem to be heading in the direction of a cause and effect relationship. The connection between boxing and classic CTE is solid and doubted by few. The connections between repetitive mild TBI, concussions, and clinical modern CTE are less well accepted. There is great interest in this area, and research is not only ongoing, but expanding. There will be more forthcoming.

The revelations about Thomas, the incidence of this disease among NFL players, and the heightened awareness about concussion in general, led Paul Davies, the deputy editor of the Philadelphia *Inquirer*'s editorial page, to question whether playing football is worth the risk. In a commentary dated September 19, 2010, just five days after the Owen Thomas story appeared in the *Inquirer*,

Davies questioned the wisdom of parents allowing their children to play this game.

"I understand," he writes, "why a pro football player would run back on the field minutes after suffering a concussion. The answer is money." But given the vanishingly small chance that any individual peewee football player has of an NFL career, does it make any sense, Davies wonders, for a parent to expose a child to the thousand little hits that start at the youngest ages of competition?

Awareness of this danger has even made it into popular culture. In November 2011, the television show *Harry's Law* dealt with this problem. The show's lead character, played by Cathy Bates, is a fictional lawyer known for taking on hopeless cases. She agrees to represent the parents of a high school football quarterback who dies after a seemingly routine hit. The court case highlights much of what I have discussed in this chapter, including a straightforward lay summary of the research into CTE, cumulative brain trauma and sub-concussive injuries. The writers and actors do an excellent job of portraying the heartbreak of this fictional family.

Unfortunately, for Owen Thomas' family, and for too many other real families, the heartbreak isn't fictional. It's very real. It may be time to revisit the 1905 concern about football. The game is far too institutionalized in American culture to ever consider banning it. That case is also made in the *Harry's Law* episode. But following the example of Teddy Roosevelt, more thought needs to go into improving the safety of the sport.

Life imitates art. There is currently a lawsuit winding its way through the courts that pits NFL players against the NFL. In it, the players accuse the league of intentionally hiding information they had about the pernicious nature of the head injuries the players were sustaining in order to protect the multi-billion dollar business that is the NFL. The owners argue that player contracts cover disputes between the sides, and therefore that they should not be heard in a court. The players counter with the argument that the contracts do not cover fraud and negligence on the part of the league, which is what they allege the hidden information constitutes.[22]

As of April 2013, there were 4,200 plaintiffs in the class-action suit, consolidated from several hundred individual suits. I think the players may have a point. In 1982, shortly after I finished my residency and started in practice, a senior orthopedic surgeon on staff at my hospital, who was also the team doctor for the local NFL team, asked me if I wanted to be the neurosurgical consultant to the team. I was flattered and looked forward to being involved with the celebrity athletes. I told my colleague that I took a pretty hard line when it came to concussion. (The term TBI wasn't in common usage at that time.) I would not send a symptomatic concussed player back into the game, and I didn't want the coaching staff to override my recommendations. After all, I had just graduated from one of the premier neurosurgical training programs in the country that was also one of the nation's few NIH grant-supported head injury treatment and research centers. I thought I had some credibility.

Not so. My career as an NFL consultant was very short-lived. I never heard another word, never attended a game or saw a player. To this day I don't know who replaced me, if anyone, and that experience leads me to believe that the management of the league did not want any sticky gears slowing their moneymaking machine. Now, thirty years later, the information has become too pervasive and convincing to ignore. The players realize that their best interests may have been secondary to the interests of the owners, and that thousands of their fellow athletes are now paying the price for that decision.

One of the arguments made by the league, and it's also a valid one, is that the players knew about the inherent dangers of long-term participation in contact sports. There were many examples of their peers and predecessors who suffered cognitive problems in later life, and everyone was aware of the fact. Boxers, as mentioned, even had a name for it. It's therefore self-serving, say the owners, to claim that the league intentionally hid information from the players. The information was public knowledge (the research did not come from NFL sponsored studies that they could hide), and the NFL Players Association had as much responsibility for being aware of and disseminating the information as did the league.

Additionally, NFL-caliber football players do not come by their talent late in life. These world-class athletes start their football careers in childhood and play at every level of competition starting as early as the pre-teen years. The opportunity for sustaining concussions exists from the earliest periods of play, and it's unlikely that a single professional player sustained his first TBI in the NFL. And as we're learning, the injuries sustained early in life likely play a larger role in setting the stage for later brain dysfunction than those injuries that come in the more mature brain. Why then, argue the owners, should the NFL be singled out? The "blame" for the neurologic decline of so many retired pro football players is widespread and includes the players themselves.[23]

The league's argument is valid. But as is common in tort law, the liability tends to rest with the offending defendants that have the "deepest pockets," that is, the greatest ability to pay an award. Pee Wee leagues, public schools and club football teams do not fit that description. Universities do to some degree, but the NFL is wealthy in the extreme and is the obvious target. And the fact that other institutions are also at fault does not absolve the NFL of its contribution to this health problem.

The public has a right, and a need, to be fully informed. There has been no informed consent. The situation has begun to improve due to the accumulating volume of information about concussions that has become known to the general public and in the medical literature, but that came too late for Owen Thomas and the current NFL alumni who suffer with CTE. If the NFL had long-term knowledge of the problem and willfully withheld it from players as the lawsuit alleges, then there's little question about their part in this. It places the NFL in the same position as the tobacco industry, which was proven to have buried data regarding the dangers of smoking.

On August 29, 2013, the NFL and the players' union reached a settlement in the lawsuit. Included in the deal is $760 million; $675 million in compensation to eighteen thousand retired players, $75 million coverage for medical exams, and a $10 million commitment to underwrite research into head injury. The terms also stipulate that the settlement is not an admission of guilt by the league.[24] But there may be a problem with the agreement. In a follow-up to his August 29 article, Ken Belson reported that the number of former NFL players eligible for compensation may be far smaller than eighteen thousand. In a confidential letter sent October 9, 2013, to one of the law firms representing the players, it was revealed that only players with the most severe injuries would be compensated; the families of those players who died before 2006 are excluded. Payment would be based on the athlete's age, illness, and the number of years he played in the NFL.[25]

On January 14, 2014, District Judge Anita Brody rejected the initial $765 million settlement, claiming that she felt the amount was too low to provide adequate compensation to the players. She wants more time to examine the facts that led to the determination of the settlement amount. She also cited an apparent effort to protect collegiate football programs from similar lawsuits.[26]

Strong regulation of the participation of children is necessary. Banning organized tackle football for children under sixteen would be appropriate. Not to do so would be a sad indictment of us as parents and adults with responsibility to embrace change as new information becomes available. Close scrutiny of those between sixteen and college age, essentially high school football, is necessary. If studies show ongoing danger to this age group, strong measures will be equally necessary. At the least, parents of children participating in tackle football need to be aware of this information, and clear and easily understood consent forms should be required of all football programs.

I've discussed what is required of a surgeon in informing a patient about the risks and benefits of having surgery. The same can and should be provided for the families and participants in contact sports. Far more parents will likely be unwilling to allow their child's participation if appropriately informed.

When I was in eighth grade, I was a receiver on my junior high school football team. I wanted to continue playing on the high school team the following year, but my parents would have none of it. I was forbidden from even trying out. I was angry and embarrassed by my overprotective parents overstepping what I thought were reasonable boundaries. The knock that my and later generations get for being "helicopter parents," parents who hover over their children and obsessively protect them from any conceivable danger, can be explained by similar parenting of the previous generation.

Little did I know how prescient they were. My parents were well educated but knew none of what I've explained here. In retrospect they just knew intuitively that throwing my average-sized frame against others of any size was not a wise health choice.

"Play golf, or tennis," they said.

I did. You know how that worked out.

Nothing I've said in this chapter will be popular in Texas, where high school football is something of legend, memorialized in a book, movie, and television show. I don't care. Every parent in America who has a child who wants to play football should have this information, and as we learn more, it's going to get increasingly difficult to balance the two competing desires—the one to play the sport and the one to protect our children.

And it's not only football. Rugby, soccer, lacrosse, skiing, and every other sport you can think of, where the head, and particularly the immature head, is prone to the "one thousand little hits," will eventually be part of this story.

As disturbing as these revelations are, the story gets worse—head injuries don't only affect the head. Amyotrophic Lateral Sclerosis, or ALS (popularly known as Lou Gehrig's disease), is a degenerative neurologic disease that affects the motor neurons of the spinal cord. It is a relentless disease that slowly but progressively robs the patient of the ability to use his or her muscles. Weakness and loss of coordination herald the onset, followed by muscle atrophy, spasticity, involuntary twitching, and, finally, eventual paralysis. The respiratory muscles are also involved, so death is by slow suffocation complicated by recurrent pneumonia.

It does not affect the brain, however. So the afflicted patient remains fully aware of what is happening up to the very end. It can take variable forms. In most cases, ALS runs its course in a few years, two on average, as it did with Lou Gehrig, whose name has become synonymous with ALS. In other cases it can be indolent, and even stabilize, as it has famously done in the case of Stephen Hawking, a world famous physicist who exemplifies the fact that the intellect is unaffected by the disease.

There is no treatment, and the cause is unknown. There are recent findings, however, that point to repetitive head trauma as a cause in some cases. If this information is confirmed, it suggests there are two different forms of ALS, a form of motor neuron disease (MND). And if so, Lou Gehrig may not have had the more classic spontaneous type. Gehrig had multiple head injuries in his athletic career, raising the possibility of an alternative explanation for his disease. We will never know, however. Gehrig was cremated.

The evidence comes from a 2010 study published in the *Journal of Neuropathology and Experimental Neurology* by authors Ann McKee, MD, and Robert Cantu, MD, from the Center for the Study of Traumatic Encephalopathy at Boston University.[27] They showed that there are two proteins found in the spinal cords of athletes who are diagnosed with ALS. They have the classic symptom complex described above, but these proteins were not previously found in the spinal cords of those with the classic form of ALS. They are, however, found in the brains of athletes with CTE.

McKee and Cantu have named this particular ALS-like form of MND "chronic traumatic encephalomyelopathy." They reference a recent study that showed an incidence of ALS in more than seven thousand professional Italian soccer players six-fold greater than expected. They studied the brains and spinal cords of twelve deceased athletes diagnosed with CTE: seven football players, four boxers, and one hockey player. Three of them—two football players and one boxer—had been diagnosed with ALS in life.

All twelve brains showed a build-up of tau, a protein found in the brains of CTE patients. The unexpected finding was discovering the same tau protein in the spinal cords of the three athletes who had suffered from ALS.

Tau is not a feature of classic ALS, leading the authors to the conclusion that this was a new form of ALS; in fact, a new disease.

A second protein, TDP-43, is commonly associated with neurodegenerative diseases, including ALS. TDP-43 was found in ten of the twelve brains with CTE, including the three with ALS. In those same three spinal cords, TDP-43 was also found, as it is generally, in ALS patients' spinal cords. McKee and Cantu conclude that it's possible that "a distinctive widespread TDP-43 proteinopathy is associated with CTE," and if it spreads to the spinal cord it "is clinically manifest as MND."

This is all very preliminary information. The number of brain and spinal cord specimens examined is small, and our understanding of tau and TDP-43 is incomplete. It will take a great deal more data-gathering by these investigators and confirmation by others, before this information can be considered definitive. But it does represent an intriguing possibility as a means of understanding the link between repetitive head trauma, and what is clearly its clinical effect on brain function. The added possibility that the spinal cord is equally vulnerable, even in the absence of direct spinal cord injury, is of concern.

What exactly are we doing to ourselves, and our children, when exposed to those one thousand little hits?

In response to this rising tide of information about the dangers of even minor head injuries, especially if they are repetitive, many states have now enacted legislation dealing with the issue. On November 9, 2011, Pennsylvania became the thirty-first.

The law, the "Safety in Youth Sports Act," went into

effect on July 1, 2012. It mandates that any student athlete concussed while participating in a sport be immediately removed from play for the remainder of the competition. It covers game day, practice, scrimmage, and cheerleading. It pertains to public schools and club sports. Private schools are not covered by the law but in general have voluntarily followed its provisions.

Coaches are required to obtain yearly certification by completing an on-line educational course. They are schooled in recognition of the signs and symptoms of concussion, and its emergency treatment. They are not allowed to return the student to play at any level until the injured athlete is entirely symptom-free and has been cleared by an approved medical professional trained in the care and evaluation of mild TBI.

Once cleared, there is a five-step program to reintegrate into participation. It starts with simple exercise excluding running, jumping, or any jarring activity. The level of exertion gradually increases provided that at each step there is no return of symptoms. If symptoms do recur, the student returns to the last step where there were none and starts again. The fifth step is full contact practice after which, if tolerated, return to play is permitted.

Violations of the law carry severe penalties. After the first violation, the coach is suspended for the remainder of the season. After the second, suspension is for that season and the next. Permanent suspension from coaching follows the third violation.

I have been caring for concussed individuals of all ages for my entire career. Many physicians, especially pediatricians, see such patients when the injury occurs in one of their established patients. If the concussion is anything other than the most mild, the patient usually is referred to a neurosurgeon. The new law, however, requires that the medical provider clearing an injured student to return to play be trained in TBI. What that training entails is not specified. My concern is that some physicians, previously willing to care for injured student athletes but without specific training, will balk after passage of the law.

In response, the Neurosciences Institute of my hospital, which I chair, developed a concussion evaluation service. It was conceived to provide expedited access to participating physicians in order to clear the student to start the return process. Part of the service is educational, and we have provided programs to coaching staffs, trainers, parents, and students at several of the high schools in the area.

Since its inception in September 2012, we have seen and evaluated an average of forty concussions per month. The number is increasing as we've visited more schools, and as the awareness of the program has increased. We have also presented to family practitioners and pediatricians, further widening the referral base. As is to be expected, more non-sport, non-student related concussions are being sent to us also.

Later in this book, I will discuss how some sports, skiing in particular, have made serious strides in improving safety. For many sports however, the culture has been to avoid change rather than embrace it, and serious discussions of the dangers of a sport are only recently being heard; the NFL lawsuit for example. As a physician who treats the damage of sports, I know that fail-safe prevention is not achievable. As long as heads collide with other objects, there will be brain damage.

Boxing should be banned. Banning scholastic football isn't out of the question either. One high school football coach I met when invited to speak to the school's coaches about concussions reacted wistfully to the new rules that came with the state concussion act. He has already seen lawsuits filed as a result of high school football injuries. His opinion was that within ten years, the liability of a football program would be too much for a school district to bear. His wistfulness, I came to realize, stemmed from his conviction that high school football isn't long for this world.

The liability issues may be what will ultimately determine the fate of non-professional football. Changing deeply ingrained behavior can be both difficult and painful. The voluntary cessation of contact scholastic sports is a concept that is in its infancy. Banning football will pit the right of the individual to choose a lifestyle against the right of a poorly informed child to be protected from unnecessary danger. I doubt there is a politician alive who is willing to spearhead that cause. It is up to the educators, therefore, to get out the word and make sure there is informed decision-making.

HOCKEY

Behn Wilson is a large man. I met him in 1983 when Pam and I finally decided to make the move to the suburbs. We had been living in University City, a section of West Philadelphia that is in close proximity to the University of Pennsylvania, where both of us worked. Many of the inhabitants of the area similarly had some connection to Penn.

Our first child was a year old, and we thought, as did many of our generation starting careers and families, that it was time to trade urban congestion for grassy backyards and neighbors whom we couldn't hear through a shared common wall. We moved to Bryn Mawr, a toney neighborhood with what is considered a very desirable zip code. Home to Bryn Mawr College and close to Haverford College and Villanova University, the town sits right in the heart of the Philadelphia Main Line, a series of towns west of Philly along a train route that was once called the main line. We bought a newly constructed home that was more than we could comfortably afford, assuming my future earnings would make that situation short-lived. Virtually all of the families that moved into that neighborhood were in the same stage of life.

Behn and his family were among them. A bit further along the line in financial comfort, he was an NHL star defenseman. He played for the Philadelphia Flyers from 1978–83 and the Chicago Blackhawks until 1988 when he retired. Behn was a strong, tough skater and never shied away from an on-ice brawl. He was in fact known for being fearless. While a member of the Flyers, the team was known as the "Broad Street Bullies," named for the street the stadium was on, and he was the persona of the team. Off the ice he was the exact opposite: gentle, quiet, intellectual, and a loving husband and father to his three daughters. He was one of three professional athletes who lived in the neighborhood and shared a similar disconnect between their public and private personae.

It was Behn who reminded me that it was possible to have a concussion of the spinal cord. During a game while playing with the Blackhawks in 1986, he was checked by an opposing player. He flipped up into the air and landed on the ice flat on his back. He was rendered instantly paraplegic, unable to move his legs, and anesthetic from the chest down. He was taken off the ice on a spine board and admitted to a hospital. An MRI scan was normal. Within a few hours, he was moving his legs and over the next days he recovered fully.

I was unaware of his injury at the time. Behn and his family lived in Chicago during the hockey season so there was no buzz in the neighborhood, and I never saw anything in the Philadelphia press. He didn't play for the remainder of the season, and when I next saw him in the neighborhood, Behn discussed the details with me. He was appropriately worried about what it meant for his future and what risk he ran if he continued to play. I wasn't really sure. It was my first experience with this kind of injury, but intuitively it had to be a concussed spinal cord.

It followed the familiar pattern of cerebral concussion: head injury—immediate loss of neurologic brain function—slow, gradual recovery; spine injury—immediate loss of neurologic spine function—slow, gradual recovery.

I used that reasoning to advise Behn that there was some increased risk of sustaining a second spine concussion with a lesser injury, but after only a single injury, he could return to play once all the symptoms had completely resolved. He did play the following season, but sat out the next and then retired. The last time I spoke to him he was fine, but we've lost touch since I moved from that home, so I don't know if there were any late-term consequences.

Spinal cord concussion (SCC) is far less common than cerebral concussion. The first description appeared in 1879, and in the 135 years since, fewer than two hundred cases of SCC have been reported in the English-language literature. The majority are sports-related, mostly in football. Approximately 2 percent are hockey-related. The classic presentation is associated with forced flexion or extension, or axial loading of the cervical spine with the injury at that level of the spinal cord. The loss of function is brief and can involve any or all of the limbs. Imaging of the spinal cord is normal, although there can be evidence of associated bony or soft tissue injury. There have been reports suggesting preexisting congenital stenosis, or narrowing of the spinal canal, which predisposes an athlete to this injury. The presence of stenosis, however, is not seen universally in SCC.[28]

SCC is classified based on the degree of functional loss and the time to resolution of the symptoms. It can be plegia (complete motor loss), paresis (incomplete motor loss) or paresthesia (motor intact, presence of tingling); Grade 1 (less than fifteen minutes), Grade 2 (fifteen minutes to twenty-four hours), or Grade 3 (longer than twenty-four hours). Deficits lasting longer than forty-eight hours are likely more severe than concussions and frequently leave some degree of permanent loss of function.[29]

There is a similar but more pernicious injury described primarily in children called SCIWORA—Spinal Cord Injury WithOut Radiographic Abnormality. Coined in 1982 by Pang and Wilberger, the term describes a spine injury, usually cervical, in which there are no radiographic findings of bone injury or malalignment.[30] It is often a non-sports related injury. The confusion between this and SCC comes from the fact that the term refers only to standard x-rays and CT scans (which are also created with x-ray). Unlike SCC, MRI scans in SCIWORA are uniformly abnormal and show ligamentous and spinal cord injuries that cannot be seen on CT and x-ray. MRI scans are created using magnetic energy and are therefore technically not radiographs, or x-rays. Since the advent of the MRI era, SCIWORA has become a less useful designation. The more accurate description of the injury as a spinal cord contusion or hemorrhage, diagnoses that can be made with MRI, are far more useful and predictive of eventual outcome. These injuries are almost always associated with permanent neurologic deficits.

Statistics from different reporting entities vary, but the Center for Disease Control estimates there are approximately 1,500 sports-related spinal cord injuries per year in the US. They are most common in contact sports, diving, and equestrian sports. The mechanism of the injury is forced flexion or extension of the neck by a force applied to the vertex of the head.

In serious SCI, there is loss of the normal spinal alignment caused by fracture of the vertebral body and disruption of the ligamentous support structures. Fracture-dislocation is the classic description of this injury.

The translational motion of the destabilized segment traps and injures the spinal cord housed within the now unstable spinal column. The injury to the cord in this setting is usually catastrophic and permanent. The athlete experiences immediate paralysis that can be either partial or complete. In cervical spine injuries of this type, all limbs are affected—quadriparesis (partial paralysis) or quadriplegia (complete paralysis). Thoracic-level spine injuries are less common because of the support added by the rib cage and the bulk of the trunk. When they do occur, only the legs become weak—paraparesis or paraplegia. The cervical spine is less protected and far more mobile, accounting for the bulk of the injuries being at this level.

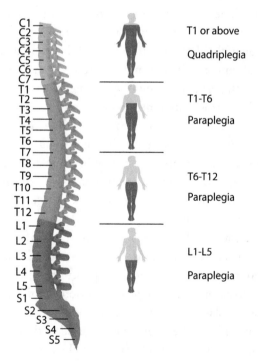

Spinal anatomy.

Lumbar injuries too are uncommon for similar reasons. Although there are no ribs supporting the lumbar spine, the bulk of the trunk and limited flexion and extension in this spinal region protect it from injuries. There is no spinal cord in the lumbar spinal canal. The cord ends at the thoraco-lumbar junction. Below that level there are only nerve roots that have the appearance of a horse's tail and take the Latin name for that structure, the cauda equina. The rare injury to the lumbar spine can cause a wide variety of different neurologic deficits depending on which and how many of the roots are involved.

The usual contact precipitating an SCI in football is tackling with the head or face forward. In diving or a fall from a horse, the head striking the pool bottom or ground takes the brunt of the impact, forcing the flexion or extension that initiates the anatomic failure and producing the damage to the cord. Most commonly the cord is severely contused, with a component of hemorrhage that creates the irreversible neuronal neurotmesis, a degree of injury that cannot recover. The commonly referred to "severed cord" is quite rare. The outcome can be as if it was severed, but that degree of disruption is unlikely.

Organized football at all levels of play has made an effort to minimize the incidence of these rare but disastrous injuries. It is now forbidden to tackle by leading with the head, the so-called "spearing" tackle. Unfortunately, outlawing something doesn't always eradicate it. Unintentional spearing happens on a routine basis, and rarely does an NFL game finish without at least one penalty for this infraction. The same injury can occur by the head striking other areas of an opponent's body, most commonly the knee. For all the times this potentially injuring mechanism occurs, the actual injury's incidence remains thankfully low. It is life altering and occasionally, life ending.

Chapter 4

EXTREME EXERCISE

EXTREME SPORTS & MARATHONS

In 546 BCE, Persia invaded Ionia, in Asia Minor. Ionian Greeks, a significant proportion of the Ionian population, rebelled against the Persian invaders under whom they felt oppressed. The Greeks came to the aid of their Ionian countrymen, and thus began the Persian Wars, lasting from 499 to 449 BCE.

In 490, the Persians under King Darius' generals landed at Marathon, in Greece, with some twenty thousand troops. Others put the number at seventy thousand.[1] The Greek army was commanded by Miltiades, an Athenian who had lived in Persia for many years and was familiar with their military tactics. They numbered perhaps ten thousand troops, unable to swell their ranks because Sparta refused to send reinforcements in a timely manner. The Greeks responded by surrounding and defeating the Persians, a turning point in the war.

This was the first Greek victory against their Persian adversaries. Miltiades realized, however, that as the Persians retreated to their ships they set sail not for Persia, but for Athens.

In order to announce the victory in Athens and to prepare the city for the impending arrival of the enemy, Pheidippides, a Greek messenger, was tasked to take the news of the victory and Persian approach back to Athens, a distance of approximately forty-two kilometers, or twenty-six miles, a shorter distance than the sea route the Persians would need to navigate to reach Athens. Pheidippides was not a random choice. He was an Athenian herald, a professional runner and messenger. This was, after all, a time when there was no other way to convey urgent information over lengthy distances (why they chose not to employ horses is unknown to me).[2]

According to the historian Herodotus, this same herald ran to Sparta from Marathon prior to the battle to ask for help, only to be turned down. That distance is about 150 miles and is presumed to have taken two days, not an unreasonable feat for a pro.[3] Modern distance runners can run 100 miles in twenty hours. With interspersed rest, 150 miles in forty-eight hours is not unreasonable. There is a modern race between these two cities to commemorate the battle, and the winning times are under twenty-six hours. Of course, Pheidippides had to retrace his steps to bring back the Spartans' answer.

It's unclear how long the battle lasted, but at its conclusion, Pheidippides made the shorter and more famous run to Athens. He laced up his running sandals, carbo-loaded on baklava, and set out on history's first recorded and most famous marathon. He delivered his message and promptly dropped dead.

That should tell you something.

Let's review: seasoned, professional runner, 290-mile warm-up run successfully accomplished, big battle, a few days rest presumably, chip shot comparatively short 26-mile run, dead.

And based on this, an entire athletic sub-culture has developed: long-distance running.

The marathon race is only the first in an ever-expanding line of extreme sporting events. Over the years, the long-distance run has been paired with long-distance swimming and biking in what has evolved into the modern Triathlon. This sport comes in several varieties of varying distances of the three individual events that span the spectrum from reasonable to absurd. The latter is best represented by the Iron Man Triathlon that, in at least one iteration, consists of a 26.2-mile run, a 2.36-mile open ocean swim, and is capped off with a 111.8-mile variable terrain bike ride.

For illustrative purposes, I offer the following two datelines that came from recent marathons run shortly after I wrote this chapter.

October 9, 2011, Chicago marathon. A thirty-five-year-old North Carolina firefighter collapses and dies five hundred yards short of the finish line.

November 19, 2011, Philadelphia Marathon. Two dead. A twenty-two-year-old college senior and a forty-year-old triathlete.

Headlines like this are sensational. They grab our attention and to the skeptics among us are fodder for our aversion to exercise—they're what make skeptics like me say "Aha! See? Exercise will kill you!"

Fortunately, deaths during marathons are rare. A study published in *The American Journal of Sports Medicine* in 2012 addressed mortality among marathon runners between 2000 and 2009.[4] Using publicly available racing and news databases, the authors found more than 3.7 million participants in marathon races in the US over the ten-year period studied. There were twenty-eight deaths in this number, representing only a very small fractional percentage of the total racers (.00076 percent for the purists among you).

There were six women and twenty-two men. Unfortunately, the median age of the fatalities was 41.5 years. Half of the twenty-eight were under forty-five. For those older than forty-five, the cause of death in 93 percent was as expected—heart attack as a result of atherosclerotic heart disease (hardening of the arteries). The cause of death in the under-forty-five group was varied, but the largest single reason was cardiac arrest of unspecified cause. I would surmise that this was the cause of Pheidippides' death, although I can't be sure of his age. If I could find his grave, his headstone is likely to be in ancient Greek, and I can't even read the modern version.[5]

Enough said.

As someone who has never had even the slightest desire to punish myself with such physical excess, I can't begin to understand the psychology of the motivation that pushes one to this sport. What I can do is elucidate for you the dangers involved and tell you what physiological explanation there may be for why someone would pursue such a sport.

Before I do, however, I want to clarify the name of this chapter. Extreme sports actually exist as a class. They evolved from three common items; the skateboard, the BMX bike, and the snowboard. These are ubiquitous and are seen everywhere, the first two usually being used by young males. Snowboards are so common that at many ski mountains boarders outnumber skiers. One may think participation in these activities is uncommon, but if you are a young adult, it's likely you have or still are using them. If you are older, it's likely your children are.

In most discussions about these sports, the Marathon and the Triathlon are not included among them. For the most part, extreme sports are common, well-known sporting events placed into absurdly dangerous situations. And although boards and bikes are still employed, they have moved well beyond those devices as well. Among the many:

- BASE jumping using various forms of devices to create drag, (BASE is an acronym for Buildings, Antennas, Spans-bridges, and Earth-cliffs, the four fixed objects from which one can jump.)
- Bicycling on unstable terrain such as sand, dirt, or straight downhill,
- Skiing and boarding on steep and variously shaped geometric platforms,
- Skating on concrete, asphalt, and variably designed geometric forms with hard surfaces,
- Boarding on similar surfaces when used with wheels,

- Boarding on water propelled by surf, sail, or chute, and
- Motorized land and watercraft designed to travel at high speed but affording little or no protection for the athlete.

I remember getting my first skateboard as a teenager. It was a sport with origins that go back to the 1940s, but was popularized by the California surfing craze of the 1960s, which is when I discovered it.[6] The singing duo of Jan and Dean, musically riding the crest of California surfing, released the hit "Sidewalk Surfing," putting skateboarding on the Top 40 charts. Over time I got pretty good at it. As I became comfortable with a level of boarding, I began to experiment with more challenging, and more dangerous, maneuvers. I had my share of falls with the attendant injuries, but luckily, none was serious, and before I had a bad injury, I lost interest and gave up my board.

Many others stayed interested, and gave birth to organized extreme sports. In 1995, ESPN realized the growing interest in these sports, and their value, and hosted the first Summer X Games. They included skateboarding, bungee jumping, BMX biking, mountain biking, street luging and moto cross among others. In 1997, ESPN gave us the Winter X Games that highlighted snowboarding, snowmobiling and skiing. The Games legitimized the sport and drew hundreds of thousands of spectators and viewers, along with the sponsors eager to tap this new and lucrative market.[7]

These sports are very seductive. There is a high degree of thrill associated with them, and many of the best athletes in these sports have become celebrities, especially among teens and young adults. They are heavily marketed, show up in popular magazines and on the Internet, and receive endorsements that associate these new stars with clothing, sport drinks and energy foods. Because the equipment is affordable, and, especially for skateboards and bikes, the venue is just outside the front door, kids everywhere, especially boys, gravitate to their use.

This section isn't for the rare athlete who gets on a board or a bike as a pre-teen, shows talent for the sport, and becomes good enough to make a career out of competition. And it's the rare adult who bikes or boards and still performs dangerous stunts. But every kid rides a bike. Many skateboard. Snowboards are everywhere. My children used all these; so have I. But even helicopter parents are routinely out of sight of their children. It doesn't take much to build a ramp that will launch a rider into the air over a landing spot that has probably been given very little forethought. Parents: beware.

Given the limitless nature of man's imagination and the ability to adapt sport to revenue, it wasn't long before extreme sports pushed through the boundary of extreme into the realm of the absurd. Some of the games defy intelligence. Take for example:

- Volcano boarding (self explanatory)
- Train surfing: riding or "surfing" on the top of a moving train
- Crocodile bungee: bungee jumping into water containing live crocodiles.

Then there is my favorite, Air Kicking, in which a catapult launches the participant twenty-six feet in the air into water or a foam pit, using a combination of air pressure and water recoil as the propellant. This is not new: P. T. Barnum and James Bailey called this the human cannonball. It was, and remains, a very popular circus act. What is new is that this is now defined as a sport. Ironically, the definition of circus includes references to sport and athletic events, so there is a kinship between Air Kicking and cannon balling.

The web site RationalWorldView.com, in August 2013 looked at the dangers inherent in these sports and pointed out that injuries are a growing problem that needs to be addressed. The article highlights several high profile athletes that have sustained serious permanent injuries such as traumatic brain injury and paralysis, and death. An injured dirt biker is quoted as saying spectators "want to see people go out there and crash because the crowds get excited . . . that's what the crowd loves."[8]

Extreme sports aren't only played to the extreme. They are evolving in the extreme. The sports have no governing body that provides oversight. They are getting more dangerous and the level of risk is increasing. In the first Winter X Games, the snowboard half-pipe was twelve feet tall. It is now twenty-two feet high. The Big Air Mega Ramp, which skateboarders and BMX bikers use to launch their aerial acrobatics, stands sixty-two feet high. Rational World View points out that these sports have turned the athletes into daredevils. "Spectators watch to be thrilled more than they watch for the sheer competition of the event."[9] Once again, the specter of the gladiatorial ring is evoked.

In medicine, there is a concept known as the LD-50, or Lethal Dose-50, which stands for the dose of a drug that would be lethal for 50 percent of those who ingest it. The term has been generalized to non-drug related events. An example is the height of a fall onto a hard surface that kills half of those who have such fall. The LD-50 of falling from a height is thirty feet. With the Mega Ramp at sixty-two feet, falling carries a high risk of death.

The author of the RationalWorldView.com article takes a strong stand both about who is to blame and what needs to be done. He points to the organizers and sponsors of the game who reap huge profits but fail to take into account the safety of the athletes. He calls on them to ban certain elements of the sports that carry significant danger and to cease the changes that infuse danger into the sports. "Start by ending the ever increasing height of the half pipes and super pipes."[10]

For comparison consider any number of standardized sporting equipment benchmarkers, for example gymnastic equipment such as the balance beam and the parallel bars, that have been standardized for decades. They are not redesigned every time proficiency on them is achieved. Not so with extreme sports, suggesting that changes are made to increase the inherent danger in them rather than the proficiency required to perform them. The RationalWorldView.com article concludes with a call to establish rules and parameters such as exist in all other organized sports. Otherwise, it states, it's nothing more than a thrill show, not a sport.[11]

I agree entirely. Traditional sporting events grew from the very human trait of the desire to compete and best an opponent. Extreme sports grew from a realization that they could produce wealth. If competition were truly at the heart of the games, the intentional infusion of increasing danger would cease. Like the gladiator ring of old, the extreme arena purposely places participants in harm's way. If the competitors are too immature or too blinded by the financial benefits to govern themselves, then oversight will eventually be imposed. Unfortunately, that often materializes only after public recognition of tragic events. Which athletes, and whose children will that be?

Over the past twenty years, a form of training that shares the philosophy of sport without limits has found an ever expanding following.

CrossFit is a form of extreme exercising that has been embraced by most adult age groups. The July 31, 2012, issue of *U.S. News & World Report* published an online report of this increasingly popular fitness program. It began as a form of training for the military and first responders. Over the past decade it has evolved worldwide, and there are now thousands of sites, known as boxes, where this type of training is available. As with many other forms of extreme sports, it has developed its own international games with the top athletes competing at the professional level.

CrossFit is designed to improve physical ability and agility by way of a strength and conditioning program incorporating aerobics, gymnastics and weight lifting in intense and varying combinations that change daily. The workouts of the day, called WODs, are chosen randomly and may incorporate any of the myriad exercise modalities used.

"A typical WOD may be an 800-meter run or row followed by two reps each of 22 pull-ups, dead lifts, and thrusters (full squats with a barbell and pushing the barbell overhead as you rise), ending with another 800-meter run or row. Due to the variety of high-intensity exercises, it improves both strength and endurance while enhancing accuracy, agility, flexibility, and more. WODs are never boring and they're quick, lasting anywhere from five to 30 minutes."[12]

The author of the article extols the positive affect CrossFit has had on her. The other attendees of the box where she exercises have become her "second family." There is a great camaraderie that had developed among them. "It's a fun, exciting, and challenging way to exercise that's scalable for everyone, regardless of age, sex, or athletic ability."[13] Included in its many positive aspects are weight loss, boosted metabolism, and improved blood pressure, blood glucose, insulin levels and cholesterol.

Seven years earlier, Stephanie Cooperman painted a very different picture of CrossFit. In a *New York Times* article entitled "Getting Fit, Even if it Kills You," she relates the story of Brian Anderson, a member of the Tacoma, Washington sheriff's special weapons and tactical team.[14] After a particularly stressful thirty minute CrossFit workout, using a forty-four-pound ball with a handle that allowed him to swing it in arcs from overhead down to between his legs, fifty times, take a short rest and repeat fifty more times, he had such bad back pain he couldn't walk. The pain worsened, and later that night, in a hospital emergency room, he was diagnosed with rhabdomyolysis.

Rhabdo, as medical personnel call it, results from the sudden, widespread breakdown of muscle fibers, leading to the release of fiber cell contents, primarily the protein myoglobin, into the bloodstream. If enough myoglobin is released, the kidneys can shut down causing acute renal failure. There are several possible causes; severe exertion is one of the well known ones.

Anderson spent six days in intensive care. An Army Ranger prior to entering law enforcement, he recovered fully and six months later returned to the CrossFit training that almost destroyed his kidneys, stating "I see pushing my body to the point where the muscles destroy themselves as a huge benefit of CrossFit."

Cooperman points out that this particular brand of exercise is a set up for injury, especially for beginners who may be poorly supervised. Emphasis is placed on speed, weight and quantification of results in the form of number of repetitions, weight lifted and time of participation. She quotes Wayne Winnick, a sports medicine specialist from Manhattan, as saying that "There's no way inexperienced people doing this are not going to hurt themselves." Even the founder of CrossFit, Greg Glassman, told Cooperman "It can kill you, I've always been completely honest about that."

She continues with a back-and-forth dialogue between supporters and critics of CrossFit. Gym owners express concern that when they show up in groups, these extreme exercisers take up too much space and over stress the equipment, leading to breakage of the apparatus. One owner worries that the philosophy of the training method, stressing speed and repetition, ignores form, leading to injury. Glassman counters the naysayers by pointing out that the intensity of the workouts act as a pre-selection process, separating the weak-willed from the gung-ho. Quoting Glassman, "If you find the notion of falling off the rings and breaking your neck so foreign to you, then we don't want you in our ranks."[15]

Unlike extreme sports, where there can be no question that aerial acrobatics at extreme heights can cause injury, there may be some element of lack of awareness when it comes to the dangers of CrossFit. This is especially so for the novice, who may see this training as a fast track to great fitness. I've always thought there should be a basic trust of those who instruct and monitor physical activities. Coaches should teach the correct way to play a sport. Referees should insure safe performance. A personal trainer should know the limits of those he or she trains and should stop short of the point of injury. I may be naive. With opinions like Glassman's, being informed is more important than ever.

I've never understood the appeal of these sports and have never had any desire to participate in them. Given my risk-adverse personality, they've never made any sense to me, and I have harbored doubts about the intelligence of those who are involved. That is particularly so for CrossFit training. I understand thrill seeking. We all do that at times in our lives, especially when young. But there is a spectrum of danger associated with the thrill, and most of us endeavor to stay at a reasonable, relatively safe point on that spectrum. We occasionally drive too fast or jaywalk, and for the adventurous, walk under ladders. Why do some people like to push the limits and engage in an activity that exposes them to considerable danger on a regular basis?

It certainly makes no sense from an evolutionary point of view. We've already discussed the biologic imperative that drives us to survive, mate, and reproduce. The survival of the species depends on such behavior. We are hard wired to avoid situations that may render us disabled, or kill us. If some of us are wired a little differently, or if there is something that short-circuits the wiring, it might explain why someone would be willing to launch himself off a ramp, somersault while riding a child's bicycle, and land on a rock-solid surface.

Joachim Vogt Isaksen wondered the same thing. He published "The Psychology of Extreme Sports: Addicts, not Loonies," In the November 2012 issue of *Popular Social Science*. He cites an interview study of fifteen extreme athletes who had similar feelings about their experiences. They related their participation in their sport to personal transformations that had positive effects in other areas of their lives. It turns out that there may actually be a physiological reason for pursuing extreme sports and exercise.

The people who seek out these dangerous sports do so because they enjoy them. It seems counterintuitive to get joy from danger, but repetitive exposure to the danger reduces the fear response and explains why the half-pipe pipes and boarding ramps get higher. Neurophysiologists have learned a great deal about the neurochemistry of the brain in recent decades. Dopamine, a ubiquitous neurotransmitter, is one of the best studied, and its release is increased by extreme experiences. It is postulated that this release creates optimism and happiness. "Dopamine plays an important role in the reward and motivational systems in the brain, and high levels of it lead to feelings of well-being. Therefore one may conclude that the effect of overcoming fear may lead to positive psychological outcomes."[16]

Isaksen suggests that surviving the dangers of these sports is akin to surviving a serious illness or accident. Such experiences can change lives and increase the appreciation of life. So too can these sports. If this is mediated by dopamine, repeatedly released into the brain by surviving a dangerous sport, it may actually be addictive. "The brain will not differentiate between the degrees of safety of the activities you perform, whether it is bungee jumping or whether it is the state of being in love. What is important is whether the activity results in the release of the nerve signals involved in the brain's reward system."[17]

It is analogous to the endorphin effect of long distance running. Endorphins have been implicated in the 'addiction' runners develop to the sport and explain why they feel ill when they miss a run; they are withdrawing. The difference is that in the case of endorphins, the effect is the result of the sport itself. In the case of dopamine, it is the fear and danger that triggers the neurotransmitter's release. It makes me wonder if extreme sport is a misnomer. It's really little more than extreme thrill seeking.

PARKOUR

Parkour and free running are two very similar sports that involve using only the human body propelled through space by running, jumping, climbing, vaulting, rolling, falling, flipping, sliding, hanging, dangling, and swinging on, over, under, down, from, through or around objects in your environment. Speed and agility are essential to the sport, which requires the participant to negotiate any passage in the quickest and most efficient way possible.

Purists of parkour differentiate it from free running primarily on philosophical grounds. Parkour considers itself an art form as much as a sport, building on Eastern martial arts, many of which imbue their sport with spiritual and lifestyle elements. Châu Belle, one of a group of practitioners who in 1997 founded the group Yamakasi, a Congolese word meaning "strong spirit, strong body, strong man, endurance," explains it as a "type of freedom" or "kind of expression;" he says that parkour is "only a state of mind" rather than a set of actions, and that it is about overcoming and adapting to mental and emotional obstacles as well as physical barriers."[18] They want their athletes to incorporate these philosophical aspects of the sport not only for their own benefit, but also as a means of achieving the physical abilities necessary to be successful.

There is a move by some to keep parkour a non-competitive sport, fearing that competition would dilute its philosophical basis of being a discipline that is altruistic and promotes self-development.[19] There is something noble about that perspective. There is also a certain beauty to watching those adept at this sport moving seemingly effortlessly, almost ballet-like, as they traverse obstacles in surprising and innovative ways.

Free running is the first cousin of parkour, and has

been used—improperly, according to parkour purists—as a synonymous English translation of parkour. It has become a popular sport developed by urban teenagers, but like skateboarding and BMX biking, has a more street-like quality. The maneuvers are similar to parkour, but it lacks the philosophical dimension.

Given parkour and free running's urban focus and the youth of those involved, the scope and magnitude of the injuries sustained by participants should not be difficult to imagine. There hasn't been much published on the risks of parkour, but participants are beginning to talk about it. In a non-scientific survey made available on social media and created by a physical therapist/parkour enthusiast, 239 people had submitted answers as of 2012.

A large majority of those answering, 85.5 percent, reported having been injured in the previous twelve months, three quarters of those from a specific traumatic event as opposed to chronic, cumulative injury. The lower extremity took the brunt of the injuries—almost 60 percent—the upper extremity 18 percent, and the head, spine, and joints made up the remainder. Most of the injuries were minor with only eleven people (5.7 percent) sustaining a fracture, and 72 percent needing no medical intervention other than self-care. The most common injuries were sprains, strains, and tears.

Most of the respondents felt they could have avoided the injury had they been better trained or in better shape, and were taking steps to achieve those ends. That is the take-home message of the survey according to its author, who correctly observes that the survey could suffer from selection bias. Those answering may have been motivated to do so because they had been injured, and those without injuries less so, skewing the results.[20]

All body parts are vulnerable, not just bones. In video and still picture images I've been able to find, very few free runners use any type of protective gear.[21] Wrist, elbow and knee guards, and head protection are rarely seen. So swinging one's way through an urban landscape provides any number of inventive ways to inflict injury. I suspect dealing with skin abrasions and lacerations is a way of life for these kids. Joint injuries of the sprain and strain type would appear unavoidable, as the survey shows. Given the reflex to extend your arm to brace yourself when falling, a particularly nasty wrist fracture called a Colles' fracture seems unavoidable. The few fractures noted in the survey were not characterized. I do have personal experience treating a skull fracture that occurred when an individual attempted to ricochet his body off a brick wall. He was a youngster, and the fracture resulted from what he described as "rough-housing," but I hadn't heard of free running or parkour at the time, and didn't ask the questions that might have clarified his mechanism of injury.

I probably don't see as much of this type of trauma as my urban colleagues. I practice in a suburban county, and I've not heard that this sport is catching on in the area. I suspect, however, that if it has arrived, it might be underground. The obvious danger involved would be evident to even the youngest of participants. I can't imagine they would want their parents to know what they are doing. Some communities are considering banning the sport. Florida State University has banned parkour, which had become popular on campus,[22] and Margate, Florida, has done the same thing, banning it from public parks in the city.[23] It's possible then, that our emergency room is treating these injuries, but the patients are not telling us the truth about their cause.

SKIING

I love to ski, and I used to ski often. I started when I was a pre-teen. My parents took us the first few times. It wasn't long before my older brother Mitch turned sixteen and started driving. We lived in southeastern Pennsylvania, not exactly the heart of ski country. The closest slopes were in the Pocono Mountains, just an hour or two away, so my parents let Mitch drive us there on weekends even when they couldn't come along. It was the 1960s, a less paranoid time.

The average winter snowfall at Elk Mountain Ski Resort in Union Dale, at the northern border of Pennsylvania, is sixty inches. That is about one fifth of the average snowfall in Vail, Colorado. The temperature is also more variable, and when it rises above thirty-two degrees Fahrenheit, the snow begins to melt. It then freezes again at night when the temperature dips back below thirty-two, but instead of turning into light, fluffy snow, the slopes become a sheet of ice.

Another feature of 1960s skiing was the absence of snow-making. The technology was in its infancy, and several of the manufacturers were suing each other for patent infringement. The smaller resorts hadn't yet adopted it. That was the case in Pennsylvania, at least where my brother and I skied. So skiing the Elysian snow-covered mountains of my fantasies was exactly that, a fantasy.

In the early days, before I had acquired any proficiency in this sport, I was usually hurtling down an ice mountain, completely out of control, praying that no one got in my way and loving every second of it. Stopping often required the employment of gravity, falling before crashing into some sort of restraining barrier, but sometimes not. The fact I ever made it through high school is a miracle.

Those days were also the dark ages of ski equipment. The skis were made of wood, with no bottom coating to minimize catching on bare spots. The bindings were called 'bear traps.' There was no release mechanism to allow the foot to come free in the event of a fall. The boots were thick, stiff leather and needed to be laced up. Comfort was not high on the priority list of the boot designers, and wearing them made the term 'bear trap' an excruciating reality.

The next generation of equipment was a leap forward. The skis were contoured, had metal edges to allow gripping on ice, and the bindings were the 'step-in' style that allowed for foot release in a fall. It was equipment design that took into account the popularity and fast growth of skiing that occurred because skiing had captured the attention of the entire world.

That attention came from the accomplishments of a twenty-four-year-old French skier, Jean-Claude Killy. At the Winter Olympic Games in 1968, held in Grenoble, France, Killy won all three Alpine skiing events: the downhill, the slalom, and the giant slalom—known as the Triple Crown. Killy was only the second skier to win the three races in a single Olympics. The other was Australian Toni Sailer in 1958.

Killy was young, handsome, charismatic, and skied with abandon. His fearless racing style was all about speed, and he became an instant worldwide hero. I was eighteen and he certainly became mine. On the slopes, I wanted to be Killy, racing down the hills at blinding speed, negotiating every twist and turn the mountain could throw at me, and coming to a graceful skating stop with snow cascading off the bottom of my skis as I dug them into the snow, my gold medal awaiting.

By that year, my equipment had become as beautiful as Jean-Claude's. 'Head 360' was the ski to own, became one of the best selling skis in history, and I had a pair. They were made of sleek black aluminum, had bright yellow lettering of the 'Head' name and '360' logo, were light, flexible, with bonded edges and a plastic bottom coating. Their technology instantly improved anyone's skiing, mine included.

The boots also improved. They became plastic, lighter, far more comfortable and closed with adjustable buckles. They were easy to put on and take off. If they got a little tight as the day wore on, I would unbuckle them on the chair lift ride up the slope to give my feet a breather.

I was getting better as a skier, the equipment was improving yearly, and I was enjoying the sport more each season. Of all the sports in which I have participated, skiing is my favorite.

At college at the University of Pennsylvania, I fell in with a crowd who were as enthusiastic about skiing as I was. It was there I discovered Vermont and Colorado and came to realize that in some parts of the country, ski slopes actually had snow on them. Over one spring break I, along with a plane full of Penn students who took advantage of a cheap charter flight the school made available, went to Aspen to ski. And there I became religious. The Rocky Mountains introduced me to a type of skiing that finally fulfilled the fantasies. Huge vertical drops, deep fluffy powder, slopes that challenged even the most expert skier, daily fresh snowfalls and dream-like vistas were the norm. If there was a heaven, I thought, it had to be just like that ski trip.

Amazingly, throughout all my time on difficult ski trails, becoming ever more daring and adventurous, I never seriously hurt myself. There were plenty of falls, some of them quite spectacular, with skis, poles, hat, and goggles flying in every direction. I took the 'face plant,' a fall where one goes face first into the snow, to a new level. There were plenty of aches and pains, but nothing a few cold beers around the fire in the ski lodge couldn't fix.

The aging process, however, has caught up to my skiing. After Pam and I married, she gamely began to ski, even though she is not a big fan of cold weather. We took several trips over the years with ski enthusiast neighbors and hospital colleagues. After the kids were born, we skied with them on family trips.

It was during these years I had my two injuries.

The first came while cross-country skiing. We were at Jackson Hole, Wyoming. It can be hard to stay focused on your skiing when the Grand Tetons are the backdrop. I've been there a few times, and the views never get old. Once I discovered what *teton* means, I was even more intrigued. I was on a gentle slope that was unexpectedly icy, a ski condition far less common out west, as I've described, than those found in the east. I tumbled forward, landing with one of the aforementioned face plants on rough, granular ice.

Sandpaper would have been kinder to my face. It wasn't a serious injury, but searing is a word I came to understand intimately that day. I popped right up, aware that no bones or joints were damaged. That's when I noticed the ice had turned red. Those two clues—searing pain and bloody ice—led me to the correct conclusion that my face did not escape the injury my bones and joints had.

I vaguely remember the first description of my face employing an analogy to hamburger meat thawing and weeping. Ugly, but it wasn't anything that wouldn't heal with a little time. On-site first aid included water, my undershirt and gentle pressure. The bleeding stopped and we were on our way again, with my attention far better focused on the ski terrain. The unrelenting pain and image of uncooked hamburgers helped with that focus. Later, back at the lodge, I added alcohol as a medicinal aid—ingested, not applied.

The second injury was on a family trip to Colorado with a group of doctors from my hospital. I alluded to it briefly in the introduction. It was another injury that occurred on a slight grade. I was skiing out of the cafeteria after lunch on my way to the ski lift a short distance away. This is automatic skiing. Autopilot gets you through these times, or so I thought. My ski caught on something and threw me over the front of my skis, one of which was immobilized by whatever it had caught on.

I already described some of the disturbing sounds made by the human body during the injury process. This was one of those moments. Everyone has heard the sound of tearing fabric. Imagine that, only demonstrably louder. People near me heard it, ironically mentioning how awful it sounded as they tried to comfort me. The pain wasn't too bad. I was able to stand, and I could ski without it getting any worse. I made the instantaneous, and incorrect, diagnosis that it was just a muscle strain. Pam was far more logical in assessing the situation, and insisted I not ski, but as I said before, doctors make terrible patients.

I was wearing tight elastic ski pants and mid-calf height ski boots. This combination of external support of my lower leg allowed for the minimal symptoms and led to the diagnostic error. I spent the rest of the afternoon skiing as if nothing had happened. By the time I quit, the leg was sore, but I was dealing with it pretty well.

I got to the chalet after the last run and changed back into my regular boots. As I peeled off my ski boot on that leg, I had the first good look at my calf. It was swollen and darkly stained from bleeding into the muscle. Without the external compression of my boot and pants, the swelling worsened before my eyes, quickly assuming the shape and size of a watermelon, and the pain began to escalate with the trajectory of a missile launch.

The correct diagnosis was a torn calf muscle. I had torn it at the site where the muscle becomes the tendon that inserts into the bone. Pam, as usual, was right. It brings to mind a philosophical conundrum. If a man says something in the woods, and there is no woman nearby to hear him, is he still wrong?

The pain became so bad so quickly that I couldn't even stand, much less walk. I was carried to the car with my arms slung over the shoulders of two of my colleagues, and I hung up my skis for the rest of the trip. The pain was relatively well controlled with ibuprofen, ice, and elevation, but any movement of the foot, which stretched the calf muscle, was unbearable. Even going to the bathroom was nearly impossible.

Among my colleagues on the trip were two orthopedic surgeons, but it was Paul Angotti, a podiatric surgeon, who came to my rescue. I mentioned him briefly in the introduction in reference to this injury. Paul is an avid sports enthusiast and accomplished ice hockey player. He's the perfect person to have along on a ski trip where lower extremity injuries are common. His fortuitous presence once again speaks to something I mentioned earlier: doctors not only work with other doctors, but they share leisure time together also.

The two orthopedists were spot on with the diagnosis, but it was Paul who was prescient enough to bring a well-stocked treatment kit on a ski trip. Using several meters of adhesive tape, he created a tape splint that immobilized my foot in relation to the leg, removing all motion at my ankle. This cleverly took away all stretching motion in the calf muscle, and I could both stand and walk using crutches with very tolerable discomfort. At least I could join the group for dinners after skiing, but I spent the days mostly supine.

It took almost nine months to heal completely. My skiing ended for the remainder of the season. And I'm pretty sure that this injury set me up for the similar, if less serious, calf injury I subsequently sustained playing softball. But taking everything into consideration, I got away lucky. (I have learned not to say this to patients. They do not feel that any injury, regardless of how minor, represents any form of luck other than the bad kind.)

Not every injured skier gets lucky. As practiced by experienced skiers, skiing is a high-speed sport. Although helmets are now used with increasing frequency, they were unheard-of when I was skiing regularly, and there is no other type of commonly used external body protection. Any armor-style protection would reduce the flexibility essential to good skiing and add weight in a sport that constantly strives to reduce the weight of the equipment.

Anyone who has ever skied has seen the building at the base of the mountain with the giant red cross on it indicating where one goes if injured. The slopes are sprinkled with members of the ski patrol, those emergency medical technicians on skis who are skilled in stabilizing injuries on-site and getting the injured safely down the mountain. My uncle Ernie, who has a vacation home in New England ski country, related to me his most vivid memory of skiing: seeing row upon row of emergency sleds lined up against the side of the aid station just awaiting use. Today, ski patrols use snowmobiles, but I have no doubt they can still get you down a mountain in a hand steered sled if need be. The sleds are there for a reason.

It should be obvious that the joint and muscle sprains, strains, pulls and tears, and the bone fractures I've described in several of the sports previously discussed are just as prevalent in skiing as they are in other sports. There is no need to revisit them.

There is one type of fracture, once common in skiing, that has been significantly reduced by the improvement in equipment technology. The mid-shaft fracture of the lower leg, referred to as a "boot top" fracture (I mentioned this first in the early chapter on running), is caused when forces are applied to the lower extremity, usually during a fall, that would commonly act at the very mobile ankle joint. But with the foot and ankle immobilized by a stiff inelastic boot and fixed to the ski in a 'bear trap' binding, the weak point in the lower leg becomes the top of the boot. I have seen frightful examples of this fracture, with the lower leg at right angles midway down the tibia and fibula, the two bones in the leg below the knee. Compound fractures—those in which the broken bones protrude through the skin—were not uncommon either. Surgery was often required to repair the more serious types of these injuries, and rehabilitation was difficult, painful, and protracted.

With the introduction of release bindings, especially later designs that allowed the foot to release in all directions, these fractures declined dramatically. It is a great example of a sport that successfully responded to a safety need, and an important example for other sports. I will return to this issue in the next chapter.

I have covered head injury in depth with reference to contact sports. They certainly do happen with skiing too, as do cervical spine injuries, although the contact is usually with stationary objects such as trees, slope-side building structures, and the ever-present ground. Skier collisions are also common, especially between less experienced skiers. This potential injury has also been addressed by the adoption of technology, admittedly low-tech in nature, but highly effective. The ski helmet is now ubiquitous on the slopes. Children are required to use them at some resorts, and their parents should certainly require them. Competitive skiers have used them for decades. With time, head protection will certainly become more widely adopted.

A type of injury unique to cold weather sports such as skiing is exposure injury. Frostbite results from prolonged exposure of unprotected skin to freezing temperatures. Hypothermia, another risk of being in the cold, is the reduction of body temperature to a point at which normal physiologic functions fail. A climatologist I once met who had spent time at a weather station in the Arctic told me he never went outside without attention to the thirty-thirty-thirty rule. At thirty degrees below zero Fahrenheit, in a thirty-mile-per-hour wind, bare skin freezes solid in thirty seconds. Words to live by, literally.

Frostbite is a thermal injury caused by the effect of extreme cold on circulation. It commonly occurs to the extremities, especially the fingers and toes. These structures are supplied by small terminal arteries (those that end at the anatomic structure they supply) and have a large surface-area to tissue-volume ratio. Because fingers and toes are small tubular anatomic structures with air space between adjacent structures, cold surrounds them. The volume of a finger or toe is insufficient to trap the heat in the tissues when exposed to cold, so the temperature of the tissue drops quickly if inadequately protected.

The explanation is yet another physics lesson and has to do with the thermodynamics of heat transfer. Body heat is lost as the heat transfers from our core outwards toward our body's surface, the skin. The greater our body mass, the more heat we retain; the larger our body surface, the faster the heat can transfer to the environment. We contain heat in our core because our chest and abdomen are large in comparison to the skin covering those anatomic parts. Our digits however, have a small volume in comparison to the area of skin covering them and therefore lose heat at a faster rate than the equivalent area of skin on the trunk. There is actually an equation for this relationship, but I will spare you.

This is the reason why we can warm ourselves on a cold day by curling up. That action in-folds some of our surface area, preventing it from being exposed as a heat loss site. Covering it with clothing of course does the same thing. Conversely, stretching out on a hot day will increase the amount of skin exposed and hasten heat loss. (This is defeated as the ambient temperature rises. Heat transfer always goes from a source of higher temperature to one of lower temperature. If it's hotter than ninety-nine degrees outside, heat transfer ceases, although our sweating will still cool us.) Every dog owner has seen his pet do just that, stretch out with legs extended fore and aft, usually on a grassy area that as likely as not is also where it just relieved itself, but provides a surface cooler than its body temperature.

Other at-risk structures include the nose, ears, and chin. The effect of prolonged lowered temperature on these structures causes their blood vessels to constrict as an adaptive mechanism to preserve the heat of the blood. Blood flow to the tissue is reduced, and the endpoint of this effect is ischemia, the process in which the tissues receive insufficient blood flow. The tissue dies and becomes necrotic. If caught in time, the process can be reversed. The skin, which blanches from lack of blood, can be warmed, restoring blood flow and normal color. If not treated in time, the whitened skin turns black, and the affected area must be amputated.

This is another potential injury that can be avoided with low-tech solutions. Like your mother used to tell you, dress warmly! Proper dress, however, can be elusive, but, like boots and bindings, ski clothing has come a long way. In my teenage years, I would run out of the house in a cloth coat and blue jeans over long johns. Any socks and gloves I could find would do, and my hat might or might not cover my ears. I had my own white-skinned near misses with frostbite as my clothing became soaked with sweat and snow, and I ignored the warning symptoms.

Today there is clothing specifically designed for the cold weather athlete. Underwear is lightweight and designed to insulate. Like bike clothing, it wicks the sweat away from your skin, keeping you dry and reducing the temperature-lowering effect of evaporation. Parkas and ski pants are made of synthetic, moisture-repelling fabrics that also insulate. Ski boots are designed to retain body heat, and gloves are so improved they look like the gloves worn by astronauts on their space walks.

Frostbite and hypothermia can be avoided. There is no reason one needs to ski cold. Proper clothing will protect you. There is one caveat: as with other special-ized sport clothing, it is expensive. This is especially true of ski clothing because you need so much of it. If you want to be fashionable as well as warm, expect to spend in the thousands. And as soon as you are fully outfitted and toasty warm on the slopes, they improve the clothing. I've always had trouble reading ski magazines. Not only are the clothes shown spectacularly as worn by gorgeous people in multi-paged advertisements, but also the stories tout the new technology as the latest and greatest. The latest and greatest you just bought last year is, if not obsolete, well, not so latest and greatest.

It reminds me of back-to-school night when my children were youngsters. The highlight of the evening was always the reading program. We all wanted our kids to be great readers. I learned to read with Dick, Jane, and Spot. Not my kids. There was always the newest theory of how to make children love to read, and the schools were quick to adopt the newest techniques. There was Phonemic Awareness, Whole Language, Sub-Lexical Reading, and Phonics. It seemed to change every year, which always made me think, what about last year? Wasn't last year's reading program the greatest? At least my children are great readers and love to read. Me too, even though I learned with two fictional siblings and their dog.

The same goes for ski clothing and equipment. If you are comfortable and warm, don't worry about the magazines. And do what I did at back-to-school night. I went for the coffee and cookies and tried not to get my posterior stuck in the little chairs.

Another danger of skiing is getting injured with no one nearby to see you go down. Some ski resorts are so large that it is easy to find slopes that are unpopulated, especially so for the young and adventurous. Even not-so-serious injuries can escalate in concern if no one is there to help you and report the injury to the ski patrol. Prolonged immobility in snow will increase the risk of developing a thermal injury. A head injury causing unconsciousness or confusion will impair your ability to call for help, and if in soft snow, your ability to breathe.

Many resorts have placed cell phone towers on their property, so skiing with a phone will allow you to call for help if need be. I recommend preprogramming it with the ski patrol telephone number. The better answer, however, is always to ski with at least one other person, especially another person with a cell phone. Very simply, never ski alone. Never.

The beautiful and vibrant twenty-two-year-old daughter of friends died in a snowboarding accident that was unobserved. She had become separated from the group she was boarding with, struck a ski-lift support pole and fell unconscious into the snow well at the base of the pole. It took almost a month to find her. It is a tragic and eternally sad example of the simple rule above.

There is a reason I have dwelled at some length with this sport. I have only the fondest memories of my skiing days. I think often of taking it up again. All my equipment is obsolete and would need to be replaced, and it would be fun re-outfitting myself with the newest clothing. I am at a stage of life where the cost would not be onerous. But I am also at the stage of life where things break, tear, and strain more easily. Never one to throw caution to the wind, I am even more careful now. But as I detail above, skiing is an example of a sport that has taken giant strides in improving the safety of participation. I would never try to talk anyone out of taking it up. That emphasis on safety appeals to me. It should appeal to other sports as well. In fact, it does.

The University of Nebraska is home to one of a growing number of sites that have shouldered the responsibility of expanding the science of sports safety. The university's new Center for Brain, Biology, and Behavior, known as CB3, was highlighted in a *New York Times* article published in July 2013. The focus of the center is football-related traumatic head injuries. Dennis Molfese is the center's director. He laments the fact that despite decades of research into concussions, there is actually very little known.

One of CB3's projects is an electronic, sensor-covered mesh cap to be placed on the head of an injured athlete. It can be used on the sidelines. The goal is to be able to record objective data about the nature and severity of the head injury, to act as an adjunct to the currently used, more subjective concussion assessment tools. If research verifies the validity of the data forthcoming from the recordings, it could provide better insight to the damage caused by the injury, providing trainers and physicians with more comprehensive information as to how to deal with the athlete and the injury.[24]

Given the high profile of traumatic brain injury in football, the NFL concussion lawsuit, and increasing pressure on the N.C.A.A. to improve student-athlete safety, research like that being done at Nebraska gets a lot of attention. Molfese is well known in sports safety research. He was recruited to Nebraska to design and equip CB3. He is one of fourteen experts in the field serving on the National Academy of Sciences Institute of Medicine Committee on Sports-Related Concussion and Youth, and heads a Big Ten-Ivy League partnership studying TBI in sports.

Another of CB3's projects in development is new MRI software that measures cerebral blood flow. It will be expensive, but for NFL teams and wealthy Division I football programs, they will be dollars well spent. The MRI scanners can be used on game days to assess injuries in any body part, not just the brain. The blood flow information in conjunction with functional MRI, a type of scan that shows how specific areas of the brain respond to stimuli and actions, obtained at the time of the injury, will likely be invaluable in determining specifics of the injury that will help trainers know when it's safe to return an athlete to play.[25]

One would think that there would be consensus on the effort to make sports safer, not just for youth and collegiate athletes, but for professionals as well. Not so. In February 2013, *U.S. News and World Report* published an online discussion about changing professional football to make it safer. In "Should Football Be Fundamentally Changed to Make It Safer?" several prominent individuals were invited to give opinions. At issue is whether or not ongoing rule changes should be incorporated into the game to make fundamental changes.[26]

Four of the six people asked to join in said no, the game should not be changed. They included the director of an academic brain research center who said better treatment of the injuries and improved equipment should take precedence over rule changes. A former NFL player recommended better player education about injuries and healthy lifestyles rather than changing the game. I suspect it might be difficult to reconcile a healthy life style with the playing of a violent sport at the professional level.

Surprisingly, David Zirin, the author of two books that take to task the sporting world for the inequities and politics that tarnish it, also voted no. He is not shy about exposing the seamier side of sports. He makes the point that football is inherently dangerous, and, given the way it's played, injury cannot be avoided. Rule changes, he states, can't alter that fact. He echoes the point I make in my discussion of the pathophysiology of head injury. As long as the brain can move within the confines of the skull, there is nothing that can keep that from happening when the head is struck.

He predicts that football will see a drop in its popularity in the future, "as casual fans drift away repulsed by the violence, much as they drifted away from boxing once we saw the deterioration in real-time heroes like Muhammad Ali." He credits public education about concussions in football with influencing the current generation of parents of young children. They will steer their kids away from the sport. He notes that in the past year, one million fewer children played youth tackle football in the U.S. "The future of the sport is grim," he states, "and the more we learn, the less safe it will be perceived to be."[27]

None other than President Obama has endorsed that movement, parents keeping their children from playing football. In an interview in *The New Yorker* in January 2014, David Remnick sat with the President on Air Force One. In the background was a television tuned to an NFL game. The topic of the concussion controversy was raised, and President Obama replied, "I would not let my son play pro football. But, I mean, you wrote a lot about boxing, right? We're sort of in the same realm." He went on to make the point that there is now a great deal of information on this subject, and there should no longer be a question about the inherent danger of playing the game.[28]

I was one of those kids whose parents took me out of the game before I got hurt. But despite what I realize was a wise decision on their part, and despite the many arguments I make in this book, I confess that I like to watch football, especially the pros. I am a long-suffering fan of the Philadelphia Eagles, still waiting for our first Super Bowl win. I look forward to hanging out in the family room on game day, cheering and agonizing along with my Eagles loving offspring, and eating unhealthy food. But I cringe at the injuries, especially so as they are repeated in slow motion from a variety of angles. The endlessly repeated showing of the 1985 injury that fractured Washington quarterback Joe Theismann's leg is an image no one who has seen it can ever erase from memory.

I know it's a bit schizophrenic, arguably hypocritical, to be calling for a ban of boxing, then sitting back and watching football. In my defense, there is a difference. The goal in boxing is to injure. The goal in football is to score points. And I would have voted yes in the *U.S. News* debate. If the right rules were enforced with strong enough consequences for breaking them, football would get safer. It might cause fundamental change; there would be less violence. Let the fans decide whether or not such a change degrades the sport to the point where we lose interest. There is a parallel argument in ice hockey. The U.S. version of the professional level of that sport features fighting prominently. The European style of ice hockey does not. The talent of the Europeans rivals that of their

U.S. counterparts, as does the popularity of the sport there. The fans have not abandoned the sport. Football could learn from that example.

I am a strong believer in the power of science and research to make our lives better. I work in a profession that exemplifies that belief. And I believe it can make us safer. It certainly has in the sport of skiing. That same goal should be applied to all sports, especially for those that have inherent danger. I certainly hope that happens. You may not believe it, but I like sports, not only watching football, but also playing the ones I talk about in this book. I want them to be safe for me as well as for everyone else who participates.

Educating yourself about the dangers of sports and exercise—and demanding that those with oversight responsibility make a concerted effort to mitigate them—is the best way to protect yourself and still enjoy your pastime of choice. In the next chapter I will discuss how organized sports amasses hundreds of billions of dollars a year by cleverly manipulating its adoring public. We should require of them that they provide the very best, and very safest product.

Chapter 5

THE SPORTS-INDUSTRIAL COMPLEX

"It commands our whole attention, absorbs our very be-
ings. We face a hostile ideology—global in scope, atheistic
in character, ruthless in purpose, and insidious in method.
Unhappily the danger it poses promises to be of indefinite
duration. To meet it successfully, there is called for, not
so much the emotional and transitory sacrifices of crisis,
but rather those which enable us to carry forward steadily,
surely, and without complaint the burdens of a prolonged
and complex struggle [. . .]."[1]

You might think the quote is one of mine. It does mirror my thinking on the global and insidious nature of the
potential for injury in sport. In recognizing the dangers
and publicizing them, I anticipate being met with the
criticism that I employ hyperbole. And any attempt to
legislate modernization into the business of amateur and
professional sport to protect the public from unforeseen

danger will be a prolonged and complex struggle, as I discuss above.

But it's not my quote. It belongs to President Dwight Eisenhower and was delivered at the very end of his presidency on January 17, 1961, during the speech in which he coined the phrase, and warned against, the military-industrial complex.

Included was his warning that there was danger that came with this security. "In the councils of government, we must guard against the acquisition of unwarranted influence, whether sought or unsought, by the military-industrial complex. The potential for the disastrous rise of misplaced power exists and will persist."

The analogy with the world of sport is in the warning about the danger of an entity so powerful that it becomes uncontrollable. Eisenhower's warning was not just about a military with unlimited power, but also about the economics of the new conglomerate which bought access to and influence over the highest levels of government.

Is there a sports-industrial complex that has amassed a momentum that defies any semblance of control? Is any control needed? Exercise, participation in sports, and good nutrition hardly seem to need any governance. The belief that these things are good for you is so ingrained in us that my arguments will seem heretical. But as we know about the moon and learned from the Jedi, there is a dark side. And the dark side is not often mentioned, especially when there is such financial incentive to extol the bright side. The total amount of money generated by sport, exercise, and nutrition in the United States is difficult to know because it is reported piecemeal, but it is staggering. The

Internet site Top Business Degrees puts the total for competitive sports at hundreds of billions of dollars.[2] David Zirin, in *What's My Name, Fool?* his 2005 expose of the sporting world, puts the annual figure at $220 billion.[3] That doesn't include exercise related spending, clothing purchases, or nutritional and dietary products. And even in the economically challenged years of the end of the first and beginning of the second decades of the 2000s, the sports industry in the US employed more than three million people.[4]

John George, writing in the *Philadelphia Business Journal* on August 14, 2013, summarized the Forbes annual list of the National Football League team values. At number one was the Dallas Cowboys. Purchased in 1989 by Jerry Jones for $150 million, in 2013 the team's value was $2.3 billion, a fifteen-fold increase in fourteen years. My hometown's Philadelphia Eagles, last sold in 1994 for $185 million, ranked seventh on the list at $1.3 billion. Owner Jeffrey Lurie has seen the value of his twenty-year investment increase seven times its original value.[5]

Marketers do a dazzling job of putting all this right in front of us using every available medium. We see it on our smart phones and digital tablets, we hear it on the radio and in podcasts, and we pass by it on billboards, buses and even the occasional backside. Nowhere, however, is it more in our life than on television. TVs keep getting bigger, and their price keeps coming down. Cable access has expanded the channel choices into the thousands, and the high definition picture quality shows us clarity of detail down to the millimeter. The players and action dramatically "pop" out of the background. We see all the best plays of the day in every sport in constant replay. NFL Films gives us slow-motion close-ups of seemingly impossible physical feats performed with ballet-like grace. We are spoon-fed every detail of the star athlete's life, whether it's the success achieved at the pinnacle of a world-class career, or the shame and embarrassment of marital infidelity. There are even entire networks devoted entirely to sport, pioneered by the now ubiquitously cloned ESPN.

The sports-industrial complex has orchestrated all this with more precision than an NFL coach's game-day offensive plan. The games are presented as majestic battles in sport specific venues, most of which have been built in the last fifteen years. It was not by accident that many of these new stadiums were built with taxpayer money. In Philadelphia where I live, the issue of taxpayer funding of the Eagle's new Lincoln Financial Field raged for months in the Philadelphia *Inquirer*.

David Sirota, writing in *Salon*, exposes the hidden taxes the public pays to fund the NFL. In "The sports-industrial complex is bleeding America dry," published in February 2013, he reveals the four sports taxes we all pay. Higher taxes to fund legislative handouts for stadium construction and tax abatements, favorable tax code legislation that applies only to sports franchises, higher cable television bills because we have to pay for sports channels included in basic service whether or not we want them, and finally the higher school taxes and tuition costs that help support athletic programs that are money losers.

Sirota presents this information in the context of America still simmering in a struggling economy. He reminds us that in a period of reduced household incomes, a slowly recovering employment market and stagnant job growth, these hidden sports taxes, forced on us by the sports-industrial complex, are unaffordable. Sirota, who describes himself as a life-long Philadelphia sports fan, makes the point that while the games are important, they are not more so than other priorities that are being shortchanged.[6]

It may not seem to follow. What does an industrial complex have to do with my concern with the bodily damage that flows from participation in sports and exercise? It is simply that the value of the industry is so great that to those who benefit from it, it must be protected at any cost. And like other mega-industries that have benefited from a product that is inherently dangerous, keeping that information from the public is integral to that protection. One of the allegations in the NFL players' lawsuit against the league is that for years the league hid information about the seriousness of concussions and their long-term effects.

Informed consent. Just as the individual deserves to know the potential complications of the surgical procedure, the risk of smoking a cigarette, the dangers of climbing a ladder, or the toxicity of consuming too much alcohol, so too should that person be made aware of the potential injuries that can come from engaging in an exercise or sport that can threaten wellbeing.

We are told we too can be better, faster, stronger. Every year brings new and improved equipment—lighter road bikes, better golf clubs, scientifically engineered footwear. Like clockwork, new diets show up in health magazines and cable infomercials. Nutritional supplements, with little or no evidence, claim to burn fat and build muscle. Energy drinks that are mostly sugar and caffeine promise us more energy to help us be over-achievers. Unlike the TVs we watch this on, all this gets more expensive. We are deluged.

The improved equipment, such as the protective equipment for football players, has been designed with a genuine desire to reduce injuries. Helmet designs especially, in an attempt to reduce the incidence of concussion, have been re-engineered with the advice of medical professionals. Nicolaus Mills however, writing online for *The Guardian* in December of 2007, suggests that these improvements are in part financially driven and may actually have unintended consequences.[7]

In response to the concussion epidemic, he argues, football coaches have relied on improved equipment to protect players from the violence inherent in the sport. The head and face protection, and all the padding, are continuously updated. But, "they support a lucrative sports-industrial complex." The equipment is ever more expensive and is replaced on a regular basis. At the professional level, it's the cost of doing business. But at the college and scholastic level, it comes out of tuition and taxes. And the equipment, in association with rule changes designed to protect players, hasn't stopped the injuries. Rarely does a game go by in which trainers do not race onto the field to attend to an injured athlete, and on a routine basis, players are driven off the field or taken out of the game.

Why haven't the improvements helped much? Mills postulates that the better equipment may lull athletes into a false sense of security, believing that injury is less likely due to the new and improved uniforms. As a result, they are encouraged to play the game with even greater abandon, bolstered by a mistaken sense of invincibility. "As a result, they all too often have no qualms about turning themselves into human missiles, tackling and blocking by launching themselves at an opponent rather than keeping their feet on the ground."[8]

Our children, too, are bombarded. Even before they can talk, kids are exposed to this assault. Cameras love to focus on the fan with an infant in tow on a warm summer day at the ballpark. Pre-verbal children are like radio receivers; they absorb information in their environment constantly and are significantly affected by it. We are confronted with the pervasiveness of competitive sport and exercise: they have become an integral part of the fabric of our lives. Exercise and sport are what we are supposed to do because we're told they're good for us. They build character, give us purpose and goals, teach us competition, make our bodies stronger, and hold out the carrot that maybe, just maybe, we can be good enough to go pro. Every Saturday, pre-schoolers with absolutely no understanding of the game are running pack-like after a soccer ball. Little League baseball has kids not much bigger than the bats they're swinging, hitting softened baseballs off a stationary elevated tee. And they're there because their parents, bombarded by the same avalanche of marketing since they were children, are already indoctrinated.

Neil McNerny is a professional counselor and parent consultant. He's written a book, *Home Work, A Parent's Guide to Helping Out without Freaking Out*. In a related topic published online, he discusses dealing as a parent with the "Athletic Industrial Complex."[9] His experience began when his children's youth coaches told him that his kids were very good at the sports they played. Each child was twelve when he heard this. They suggested he should consider advanced training so they would be in consideration for college scholarships when the time came. He describes the pride he felt and also the relief that paying for college might be a problem solved.

Then he learned what 'advanced training' meant: additional sports camps, Sunday skills development and extra speed training. The implication was that this was necessary to keep pace with all the other elite athletes who were already doing this training.

"Elite athletes?" McNerny asked himself. "He was twelve years old. When did we begin designating twelve year olds as elite athletes?" As he states in the article, "My B.S. alarm began ringing." Once he began to think critically, McNerny realized that the 'elite' designation was a mixed blessing. "It's always great to hear positives about our kids. But on the other hand, going down the scholarship path might end up with more stress and less fun."[10]

As he analyzed the numbers, he learned that the chance of any high school varsity athlete getting an athletic scholarship to college was at most two percent. That's not two percent of all high school students, he emphasizes, but two percent of student athletes in all sports good enough to play at the varsity level. In the more popular sports, such as football, basketball, soccer and others, the percentage is even lower. So what were the chances that his child, a designated 'elite athlete,' would be a scholarship collegiate athlete? About two percent; in other words, there was a 98 percent chance his children's college tuitions would come from him.

McNerny details the huge industry that has evolved to satisfy the parental desire to take their kids to the next level and lists some of the more obvious ones. Summer camps, summer leagues, travel leagues, extra training, scholarship agents, and videographers. (Scholarship agents?). And then there is the high tech clothing and equipment, travel costs of the away games and tournaments, and conflicts with class time during the school year necessitating tutors.

This all comes at a price, and it can be steep. Spending tens of thousands of dollars is common. The author relates the story of one family he interviewed with a daughter possessing great soccer skills. They had spent more than twenty thousand dollars over six years on honing her talent. In the beginning of her senior year, she sustained a season-ending injury that also ended her chances for a college scholarship. The mother describes her daughter and the entire family as being devastated. The mother ruefully told McNerny that the money would have been better used if put toward college tuition savings. "Although we had some good times," she said, "I wish we hadn't gotten sucked into the scholarship vortex."[11]

I personally wonder about the psychological costs. What about the siblings who are not gifted athletes, or have no interest in sports? Watching a brother or sister excel at an activity that is associated with awards and notoriety, and watching family resources and planning revolve around that child, will make any kid feel like a second-class citizen in his or her own family.

As I have stressed repeatedly in this book: all things in moderation. McNerny still wants his children to have a vigorous involvement in the sports they enjoy. So he will send them to summer sports camps, but because of their love of the sport, not because he is chasing scholarships for them. And he will be very wary of the industry that wants to profit from the natural desire in all of us, parent and child alike, to want to achieve at the highest levels of our endeavors.

You will never hear that participating in sports, and exercising, can be bad for you. No one from the fraternity of the sports-industrial complex wants you to think that there is a downside to buying into their message. The message is so lucrative; it must be protected at all costs. It even filters down to the lowest common denominator. In addition to creating wealth, it can breed corruption of the worst kind.

In October 2012, Jerry Sandusky, a former Pennsylvania State University assistant football coach for thirty-one years, was sentenced to thirty to sixty years in prison following his conviction on child molestation charges. He had been the founder and director of the Second Mile, a foundation for troubled boys. Because of his close relationship with the Penn State football program, and its famed coach Joe Paterno, he was allowed to use its facilities for his foundation's sports camp.

It was in the locker room showers, in 2002, where he was observed sexually molesting one of the foundation's young charges. Another assistant coach witnessed Sandusky raping a young boy. Instead of stepping in to stop it and calling the police, he walked away and went to Paterno. The senior leadership of the university dealt with the issue secretly; no law enforcement agencies were notified, nor were the parents. Sandusky was confronted by the university officials but was not disciplined and was allowed to continue his association with his foundation and its youngsters until this all became public in 2011.

Former FBI director Louis Freeh was appointed as a special investigator and, in 2012, issued a scathing report blaming Paterno, Penn State president Graham Spanier, senior vice president Gary Schultz, and athletic director Tim Curley with covering up the crime in order to protect both the university and its vaunted football program, a huge money maker for Penn State. The board of trustees fired all four individuals. Paterno, widely respected and admired not only as a great football coach but also as caring mentor to his players, saw his career and reputation end in disgrace. He died of cancer in January 2012. Spanier, Schultz, and Curley were charged with several crimes including lying to a grand jury.

The National Collegiate Athletic Association levied heavy penalties on Penn State including stripping all the team's wins for the thirteen years up to 2011, imposing a four-year post-season ban, and placing the program on probation for five years. Most tellingly, the program was fined $60 million, an amount equivalent to the gross revenue of but a single year of the football program. That is a revenue stream that potentially blinded Paterno, three university officials, and the assistant who discovered the rape—five otherwise arguably honorable men—to a despicable and ongoing crime, and for nine years knowingly allowed dozens of children to be abused, all to protect a football program. In July 2013, Spanier filed a libel suit against Freeh that, as of this writing, is still pending.[12]

President Eisenhower worried about a military-industrial complex so powerful that it had the ability to infiltrate the highest levels of government and influence decision-making of those we send to Washington to act, we assume, in our interests. We've learned over time that there are any number of powerful lobbies crawling all over Washington like insects on a feeding ground, spreading money around like it was rice at a wedding, buying congressional influence sold to the highest bidder. It's so commonplace, and we are so inured to it, that it has become banal.

I would argue that the sports-industrial complex is just as insidious. It has infiltrated our minds. It influences our behavior and attitudes, and for some, has corrupted the ability to recognize the warped actions of a child rapist. It explains why cash-strapped schools will cut academic programs before athletic budgets, and why an otherwise sedate and proper suburban housewife will hurl obscenities at a volunteer Little League umpire for calling her child out at home plate. And above all, it explains why everyone everywhere believes that exercise is good for you. And it is, at least it can be. It can also harm you, and it will at some point eventually. We are all at risk, at every age and in every stage of life. That risk may in fact be worth it in order to achieve the positive effects of being active. What you need to know, however, is what the risk is, and how significant the consequences can be. You need to be in a position to give *informed* consent.

Chapter 6

WHAT DO I DO? THE GYM, GARDENING, CONCLUSIONS

Don't ask.

I exercise with a one-pound weight. I lift it with my arm extended in front of me, flex my forearm at the elbow, and bring the mug to my lips.

There are a multitude of exercise jokes. Some of my father's show up earlier in the book. I made up the one above, but query "exercise jokes" on Google and see what comes up. I got fifty-one million results. My joke might not even be original.

I have a lifetime membership in a well-known gym, franchises of which exist in virtually every large city in the country. I actually used it faithfully in the beginning for about the same six months that I used all exercise machines I've purchased. Most of those purchases, in fact, were the result of my not staying with the gym. I fooled myself into believing that the reason I quit the gym was because it was inconvenient to go there, and if I could do this at home I'd be more disciplined.

Yeah, right. You all know the truth by now. It's because I hate to exercise, fear injury, and am lazy. There were a few other things about gyms that were unsettling to me also.

THE GYM

At least it's not in first place. In 2008, the Forensic Scientist Blog published a list of the fifty germiest places in the world. Gym equipment came in forty-fifth. It's better than money, the human mouth, and Almaty, Kazakhstan. Portable toilets, monkey cages, and the Ganges River are worse.[1] Little solace. If you look at the list critically and exclude the items most people seldom if ever come into contact with—such as slaughterhouses, the Blarney Stone, and Oscar Wilde's grave—gym equipment moves up to twenty-fourth place.

When I was still at it, in the early 1990s, my gym was as much a dating scene as it was a place to work out—not that dating and exercising are incompatible activities. The women that were there to meet guys invariably had on skin-tight gym clothing which, if worn by a woman who was already in shape, was highly distracting. As I tell my now adult children, I'm old, not dead. And back then, I wasn't even old.

Then there's the sleaze factor, which is relative and different for each individual. Seeing muscle-bound gym regulars pumping iron, while watching themselves in front of mirrors and furtively glancing at the skin-tight ones, was a little disquieting. No need to mine the possibility that I might have been a tiny bit jealous. After all, I could have ordered my own steroids to enhance my workout routine in order to obtain a physique somewhere between theirs and mine.

But what bothered me the most was the sweat. There is no dearth of sweat at a gym. It is present everywhere, in startlingly copious amounts, on everyone, at all times. It got on every machine that I ever wanted to use, and it always gave me pause. Who were the last people to use this machine? Who and what have they been in contact with? Is there such a thing as a condom for an exercise machine? Back then, I always kept a towel with me and wiped down every machine before I used it. That was worthless. All it did was spread the germs around, allowed them to get into the towel and, by reusing it, carried them between machines. Most people did the same thing. In short order, every microbe in the place was on each and every machine, carried there by those of us trying to avoid exactly that.

I recently returned to a small gym in my hospital where I often spend my day in scrubs. They're perfect for a brief workout, and if I sweat them up, I can simply change into a fresh set. I was glad to see that, at least in this gym, there are spray bottles of disinfectant available in several locations along with paper towels. Virtually everyone uses it before and after using the machines. At least our awareness of the microbiology of gyms has improved.

In searching for examples of diseases transmitted via sweat, nothing definitive comes up. The hepatitis virus is shed in the sweat, but contracting it from sweat requires a break in the skin of the recipient. The worst you are likely to encounter is the cold virus, which is just as likely to be transmitted by contact with a public door handle as it is through sweat. For me, it's just the image of sliding around in some stranger's sweat on a machine where I'm not enjoying myself anyway. It reminds me of the scene in the Ben Stiller movie *Along Came Polly* in which he plays a risk-averse statistician whose profession it is to assess risk for an insurance company. While playing basketball, he collides with an opponent, and his face gets pushed into the guy's sweaty, hairy chest. Yuck.

There is, however, the potential for the transmission of communicable diseases via shared equipment. There are a host of diseases transmitted through blood: HIV, hepatitis B, C, and delta (often referred to as hepatitis D), and bacteria such as Staphylococcus and Streptococcus are among them. It would require a very unlikely set of circumstances to be infected, however. The carrier would have to be bleeding, leave some of that blood on the equipment, following which an uninfected individual would have to get on the machine within the time period during which the infecting agent is still viable, fail to wipe down the machine, have his or her own break in the skin that comes into contact with the blood left by the first person, and have the virus or bacteria enter the blood stream. It's probably more likely you'll get hit by lightning. But who thought you could break your wrist without injuring it?

Other, less serious skin infections can occur from exercise. Any repetitive skin contact with an abrading surface such as an exercise mat, pad, or handhold can thin the epidermis enough to allow entry to bacteria. The resultant infection is called cellulitis. It's associated with redness, swelling, and pain in the area of infected skin. *Staphylococcus* and *Streptococcus* are the common agents of these infections. They are common enough in mat sports, such as wrestling, that at least one manufacturer, DoubleSport, has developed an antibiotic infused line of sports clothing and mat fabric to counter this problem. (Unfortunately, the business failed, and the product never caught on.) The treatment of cellulitis includes elevation of the extremity (although it can occur on the trunk), heat, and antibiotics.

There is a rare form of cellulitis that is quite dangerous. Known technically as necrotizing fasciitis, its popular name is flesh-eating bacterial infection. Several types of bacteria, including species of the above-mentioned Staph and Strep, cause it. It occurs if the organism gets into the deeper layers of the skin and causes a rapidly developing infection involving the skin, subcutaneous fat, and fascia, the connective tissue layer of muscle. It is fatal in approximately 25 percent of those infected. You receive treatment as an inpatient, usually in an ICU, with high doses of intravenous antibiotics and systemic support for the toxicity of the infection, which can cause shock, respiratory failure, and multisystem organ collapse. Surgery to debride the infected, necrotic tissue is usually necessary as well. It's a first cousin of toxic shock syndrome, a systemic bacterial infection caused by *Staphylococcus aureus* that is associated with tampon use. These serious infections are more likely to occur in people with other conditions, including diabetes, immune disorders, recent viral illnesses, or steroid intake.

As distinct from the milder cellulitis, these dire infections are rare, and not a good reason to avoid the gym. Gyms do provide some advantage to the injury-prone, or phobic, or both. Most of the better gyms have trainers available to help participants at any level. For the novice, they are there to instruct on proper machine use and warm-up exercises to help avoid injury, and to design exercise programs appropriate for your level of fitness. It's not uncommon for some of the trainers to have advanced degrees in exercise physiology and nutrition. Knowledge about nutrition is a bonus that comes with trainers and is an integral part of fitness.

For the experienced exerciser, trainers can help identify specific areas of the body that can be isolated for concentrated attention, and, conversely, can identify whether there is something at risk. Overuse puts a body part at higher risk for injury. Asymmetric development of a muscle group puts the antagonist muscles at risk.

Group classes and individualized instruction are often available. That can help you develop an exercise routine that works for you and put you on a regular time schedule that can be built into your day. For those who do well with regular schedules, that is an advantage. In my case however, that usually provides an excuse to skip class. Nope, can't get there today. Have to see if my car battery needs charging.

Enough of the up side. This book is, after all, about the negatives of exercise. One last one related to gym use: it is expensive. These gyms are not free. I don't even know if they have lifetime memberships anymore. Mine cost $2,000 almost twenty years ago, and it's been so long since

I was there I may have used up my lifetime. It also has a new company name, and I don't even know if they honor my original contract. I do see specials advertised all the time. I suspect they are come-on deals that, like the cable companies that offer "the three pack" for $100 a month for a year, are followed by astronomical increases in fees. Look for the ones that offer a free toaster oven. That way you'll have something to warm up the Twinkies in when, like me, you give up on the whole enterprise.

And did I mention it's boring?

To appease my strong anti-gym feelings, my wife and I have bought any number of home exercise machines, including stationary bikes, treadmills, stair steppers and elastic-banded weight machines. And there have been the impulse purchases from infomercials of thigh exercisers, tummy slimmers, arm definers, butt toners, midriff melters, and pec builders. Our most recent, the Ab Circle, is a disc with knee supports and handle bars that allow you to gyrate in swinging arcs that promises to trim the waist and get rid of the love handles.

We have good intentions. We routinely use the new piece of equipment religiously for a month. Then less frequently for the next few months, then by the fourth month or so, not at all. It then becomes a storage device for hanging clothes on, or piling up folded laundry awaiting closeting, and finally gets consigned to the basement, and ultimately given away, usually to my brother-in-law, Bill Corbett. Bill, a football linebacker in college and intermittently serious exerciser, now has one of the finest home gyms in the region as a result of our cast-offs. Whenever he's in our basement, he hungrily eyes our Trotter treadmill, one of the best made out there. We can't give it to him yet, because we're storing the weight machine on top of it.

I am a terrible role model for exercise and should not be emulated. I am a classic example of the need to adhere to the axiom, "Physician, heal thyself." I ignore all the advice of those who extol the benefits of exercise, including that of my own physicians whom I see for my regular check-ups. But I have tried. I explained earlier how I am a sucker for fancy machines and TV infomercials. I've learned of late how to resist them. I go into my basement and count the number of dust covered pieces of exercise paraphernalia already accumulated there.

I've also given you the list of real exercises and activities I have tried, and their attendant calamitous outcomes. Despite them, I have returned to my bike, but in no way could my cycling be described as regular, and for the time being, I only do it on flat terrain in fair weather. I have also revisited the Trotter treadmill. It did require some dusting, and I had to move the weight machine off of it, but given the fact that even I realize that we need to keep our bodies in motion, it is one of the easier exercises to pursue. My treadmill has options for different speeds and variable inclines, and is pre-programmed with several different types of workouts, each with multiple levels of difficulty. I start at one mile per hour with no incline. I increase as tolerated, and I don't tolerate much. As soon as anything starts to hurt, I immediately quit. I've already explained the adaptive advantage of respecting bodily pain.

I make it more tolerable by reading while I walk, something that is a little annoying when I read from books.

I have to hold them flat, and if the font is small I have trouble reading with my head in constant motion. Since I started reading from a Kindle, which is always flat, and has an adjustable font size, those problems are a thing of the past. If I say I do this irregularly, however, it's safe to bet even that is a vast overstatement.

Another problem I have with the treadmill is that it is in our basement, which isn't finished. It's a regular basement—full of things we don't want to put anywhere else. There's also the washer and dryer, the heating furnaces, the cat litter boxes, and a very noticeable lack of natural light. It's just not my favorite room in the house. That would be the garage, the only room over which I am truly master. Then there's the family room, but the treadmill is large, noisy, and totally at odds with the feng shui of that room.

I do get some exercise at work. As a surgeon, I spend considerable time on my feet in the operating room. Although I am for the most part stationary when performing surgery, there can be significant physical exertion. This is especially so for some of the more complicated spinal reconstruction cases that take several hours. Performing a long segment decompression and fusion, requiring implantation of multi-level instrumentation and bone grafting, all while wearing heavy-leaded protection from the intra-operative X-ray fluoroscopy, is exhausting. I have walked out of those cases more drenched in sweat than if I had run several miles on a hot summer day, the latter being, by the way, something I have never done. I also walk a lot, through the hospital and in my office. I once put on a pedometer, a little gadget that records the number of steps you take. By programming it with the length of your average stride, it converts the total steps into a distance. Depending on the day, the number of patients I had in the hospital or in the office, I walked between 2.5 and 4 miles. Not bad for stealth exercise, which is what I call exercise performed while really doing something else. The problem is that it is frequently interrupted exercise, which is not as salutatory as exercise performed in a sustained manner. But I'll take it.

I do also help my wife with outside household chores, sometimes, and usually with a palpable degree of reluctance often apparent in my face and voice. I am not good at hiding displeasure. She is comfortable accepting my foibles, however, so long as I keep my distance when wielding any power tools.

GARDENING

Our home abounds with beautiful, lush gardens. No visitor ever fails to comment on this. There are artistically arranged flowers and bushes, a huge vegetable garden that completely sustains us during the summer, fruit trees, even an aviary for honey. Two hens provide us with eggs. For her birthdays and anniversaries, all Pam ever wants is various forms of farm implements. She has a shed the size of a small house just for them.

We recently heard from a couple who is buying a house we sold seventeen years ago. What made them decide to buy it were the gardens around the home that Pam had put in.

She is entirely responsible for the gardens. Pam can

easily spend entire days in them and be deliriously happy. I contribute little, although she frequently urges me to be more involved. It turns out it is good exercise. Pam is thin and fit. I am less so. There is the never-ending battle against the malignant vines that are trying to choke to death the trees that surround our property. These are particularly pernicious and invasive vines that seem unconquerable. Their ground level stems can get as thick and woody as a tree trunk, and the climbing vines they give off go in an endless multitude of different directions. At their worst, they can completely engulf a tree, even a large one, such that the tree is not visible through the vine's leaves. I try and keep them at bay by cutting the thick stems. This is a chainsaw activity, so I'm generally on my own. The vines are clever, however, and hide and camouflage themselves whenever they hear me firing up the saw. At least I think they do. Pam helps me find them, and then runs for cover as I approach. It is hard work. I need to climb over and through thick underbrush, bend into unnatural positions, and muscle my way through the cutting by keeping the saw stable, all the while trying to stay aware of the mayhem this tool can cause. I work up a real sweat, even on cool days.

It's not because there is any danger in gardening that I do not indulge in it more often, it's more because I am lazy. Then again, just recently, I was seeing a patient scheduled for spine surgery later that morning and asked her if anything had changed since I had seen her in the office and examined her. She pulled her gown up and showed me her lower leg. It was red, indurated (firm or hard) and swollen, with a dark, scabbed wound in the center of the swelling.

She too is a gardener. Her favorite flower is the rose. While tending them a week before the operation she pricked her shin on a thorn, not an uncommon injury among rose cultivators. This one happened to get infected, causing cellulitis spreading up her leg. Her family physician had already started her on antibiotics and leg soaks, so what I was seeing was the process already receding.

I've already described how cellulitis can be a very serious problem if the infecting organism is particularly virulent, or the individual ignores the problem. The notorious "flesh-eating bacteria" discussed earlier can start this way, and gangrene can result from the worst of it. My patient had a mild case, and it was improving. I went ahead with her surgery and she did fine.

I told Pam that evening and described what I had seen that morning.

"I have another reason I shouldn't garden," I said. "I had a patient today injured while gardening. I'm going to call it IWG, kinda like DUI, only completely different. They are both dangerous, after all. I can start a movement. I'll call it 'Mothers Against Victimization by Vegetable. MAVV.'"

"What?!" she said.

Enough said.

Then there was the Pennsylvania chainsaw massacre.

The chainsaw I use was one of those farm implement gifts. But Pam is a little afraid of it and doesn't like to use it. I do. Given the precision I have to use when cutting in the operating room, the power and freedom conferred by a chainsaw is liberating. I love it.

One day some years ago, I was cutting up branches from a tree we had taken down. They were long, not particularly thick branches that Pam was feeding across two sawhorses. She was standing to the side of one of the horses, and I was cutting from the side of the other one, a seemingly safe distance from Pam. When the branches became too short, however, I had to make the final cut in the branch from between the two sawhorses.

On one particular cut, I was coming up from below instead of the safer top down direction, and as the saw came through the branch, Pam chose that instant to reach over the top of the one we were working on. The chain caught her hand across the meaty part of her palm. Blood began to pour out of the cut in the glove she was wearing. I was terrified that I had amputated her hand, and if I took the glove off, her hand would come with it.

It is amazing how quickly thirty years of surgical training and experience with trauma can abandon you when the patient is your wife. It was a clarifying lesson on why a surgeon should never operate on family.

I did rally, however, and ever so gently removed the glove. The hand was still attached. The laceration was an ugly one, wide and jagged, just like the teeth of the saw chain. All the fingers were intact. A quick neurologic exam showed there was no loss of motor or sensory function. I piled a wad of paper towels over the bleeding and wrapped it tightly.

Emergency rooms pay a lot of attention to people who are hemorrhaging. There is an axiom in surgery, darkly ironic, that all bleeding stops eventually. Stopping it expeditiously before it stops due to exsanguination is the preferred intervention. The fact that I was well known to the staff didn't hurt either. We were ushered into a treatment room and along with the ER doctor, I had the first really good look at the injury, under a bright light, with saline to wash away the blood and pieces of her glove.

It was very ugly, but surprisingly superficial. It looked a lot worse than it was. Nothing important has been severed. No tendon injury, all nerves intact, no open arteries; just a lot of disturbing, if not particularly serious, venous bleeding. A little hemostasis (stopping the bleeding), and a lot of sutures later, Pam was as good as new.

This was a serious IWG.

Enough said.

SO WHAT ELSE DO I DO?

There are other examples, but as with those above, they tend to be infrequent. There is no real exercise I do on a regular, reliable and sustained schedule, until recently. I've replaced the treadmill with a recumbent exercise bike. It's very safe. Unless I have a stroke, I can't fall off. I can't crash into anything, get hit by a car or chased by a dog. Instead, my dogs sit and watch me with that head tilt that dogs sometimes do. It makes them look like they're thinking, "What the hell are you doing?"

The seat is low, has a back, and is on the same plane as the pedals instead of the traditional configuration with the seat above the pedals. It's actually quite comfortable, especially if you have any back problems. It has a dual cup holder for the very thirsty, side handles with built-in pulse sensors to monitor heart rate, is easier to read on than the treadmill, and is compact enough to keep in the family room so I can watch television if I'm between books. Like the treadmill, it has a computer that allows for a variety of programs simulating inclines, down slopes and variable resistance. In the four months we've had it, I've been on it two to three times a week.

There's one more thing. I recently began exercising with a personal trainer. I decided to go in this direction because of my serial failures at exercising on my own. I just don't have the discipline to stay with it. The trainer comes every week and forces me into a vigorous hour long workout. It is mostly resistance training; weights, squats, sit ups and multiple variations of gyrations that serve to contract, for twenty repetitions, every skeletal muscle I own. It was excruciating the first week. I quickly reached that lactic acid high that comes with pushing a muscle to failure. I had violated my own rule and the next three days were particularly unpleasant. But with subsequent weeks' sessions, my endurance has increased, and the pain is gone. The days after my workout are just fine now.

I'm still riding the exercise bike at the lower three resistance levels of the twenty-four available and keeping the terrain setting at flat. I ride for thirty minutes unless anything starts to hurt, at which point I stop. Leg cramps are the most common thing that ends my cycling prematurely. I've given it considerable thought, and I don't think there's any other serious damage I can do to myself in my family room. The trainer only comes once a week. Some of his clients see him three or more times and insist on every second of the hour. If he's a little late in arriving, or has to leave a little early, that's just fine with me. And he comes to me where all the germs are native to my home and not left by someone else's sweat. Time will tell if I add a second workout per week. If history serves as a guide, it's highly unlikely.

So despite all my protestations to the contrary, I do indeed recognize both the danger of immobility and the benefit of at least a modicum of exercise. That being said, I don't hide the fact that I am lazy. I've said it before. And I hate to exercise. It is an activity that I just do not enjoy, and I find it difficult to get started. It's less disagreeable once I actually do start, but the inertia induced by my dislike makes starting very difficult. I suspect, based on no scientific investigation, that there are millions of adults just like me. It doesn't mean you should be like me, how-ever. Do better than I do. Take the advice in this book and put it to constructive use. Find an exercise you like, if that's possible, and then pursue it safely. Use common sense and listen to your body. It will speak wisely.

One last thought. There are many ways to help stay healthy. We often feel we have to exercise in order to keep from putting on weight. I have an alternative idea. Don't get heavy in the first place. That's easy to say and hard to accomplish, especially as we age and become naturally less active. So I will pass on a piece of advice that a friend's grandmother gave me many years ago.

This friend comes from a line of long-lived individuals. Her parents are still living, and her maternal grandmother lived to one hundred. I remember once asking her what her secret of longevity was. Her answer was elegant in its simplicity and obvious logic.

"Don't eat too much," she said. She was a thin woman,

as are her daughter, and granddaughter. It gave me pause to think about the many people I have seen as patients. I have noticed a trend among my patients, something echoed by all of my colleagues. We are seeing many more elderly patients than we did earlier in our careers. Visits from eighty-year-olds who are still active and independent are an everyday occurrence in my office. Visits from ninety-year-olds are not uncommon either, whereas a patient this age who could actually walk into my office was at one time quite rare. And visits from active hundred- year-olds who need a back operation because their spinal stenosis prevents them from walking more than fifty feet no longer surprise me.

People are living longer. There are a host of reasons. As a physician who has seen innumerable medical advances, even within the span of my career, I credit my profession with contributing to this trend.

The realization that staying active is healthy also gets credit. That assumes, of course, you haven't killed yourself train surfing. The age group of those in their eighties and nineties predates the boomers. The oldest boomer will be a spry sixty-nine in 2014. I am instead referring to Tom Brokaw's Greatest Generation; those who fought and came of age in World War II. I discussed them briefly in the Introduction as a generation that grew up in a simpler, less mechanized and electronically indulgent era. They didn't need to make time for exercise. It was part of everyday life.

I have noticed something else about this population: They aren't as fat as the boomers and are almost never obese. Excess weight is something that is just not conducive to long life. And since these age groups can't really exercise aggressively, they achieve their ectomorphic body habitus by not eating too much. I do ask them about their eating and exercise habits, both in the present and in years past. This is a completely unscientific way to gather data, but most often their answers are that they have always been light eaters, and many never did any organized exercise. They did and still do stay active, and almost universally enjoy walking. Pam will be gratified to know that gardening is mentioned frequently.

CONCLUSIONS

When I began writing this book it was simply to tell my own story. It was both therapy and self-justification. I've mentioned that I am exercise-averse. I've also admitted that I am lazy. There is, however, a dichotomy to that fact. I can spend hour after hour in the operating room, an activity that can be arduous in the extreme both physically and mentally. There have been times, after a long day in surgery, when I've driven home in a fugue-like state, not even remembering the trip, sat in my favorite easy chair and fallen instantly asleep, not to move for several hours, before dragging myself to bed and climbing in fully clothed. I try to remember to take my shoes off.

I have the motivation and reserve energy to find the strength to practice my profession. Earlier in my career, when I was part of a two-man practice, my partner became ill, and I covered the entire practice myself for a year. I somehow cannot find that resolve when it comes to recreational physical activity. I've had my moments when

I was younger, particularly with skiing, and I still enjoy golf when I'm not the target of an errantly hit golf ball.

But when it comes to doing something merely for the sake of its health benefits, I come up with any number of creative excuses for avoiding it. Even the goal of a slimmer more fit body can't overcome my considerable distaste for exercise. My stories of being accident-prone were therefore, in some convoluted way, my justification for my bad attitude. Expressing them "out loud" to you, my audience, was the therapy that made me feel better about my foolish attitude. I am also convinced that millions of others feel exactly as I do. We are shamed into feeling bad about ourselves, because we are overwhelmed with books, magazines, TV and radio shows, and endless advertising about the great benefits of healthy exercise and a nutritious diet. With tongue in cheek, this book is for those among you who fit into that definition.

I've had many patients who have terrible pain with strenuous activity but are perfectly comfortable within their normal daily routine. Not everyone who comes to me for surgery necessarily needs to have surgery. There are often other options. The patient who can play several sets of tennis but then has to spend the next few days in bed because of back pain, has the option of giving up tennis. Some do. If tennis means a great deal to the patient, and he or she is wiling to go through major surgery in order to be able to continue to play, I can do a spine operation that will give the patient a reasonably good chance of doing so.

The more I wrote, the more this book went from being about my injuries to being a serious look at the real dangers of exercise and sport. As a neurosurgeon who has cared for many head injuries, much of what I know I have learned from my own patients. The life-altering or fatal head injuries are thankfully the minority of those I see. When they do occur, however, they destroy families.

Far more insidious are the minor head injuries that traditionally were largely ignored by the sporting community, but over the last twenty years have been shown to be of great significance, especially when repetitive, and are arguably the most serious public health issue in all of sports. Although baseball has the reputation of being the all-American sport, for several decades football has been the most popular sport in America. And it is here that the real toll of repetitive mild traumatic brain injury has been realized. The danger exists at every level of competition starting at the youngest "peewee" level of play. Those who play for a career are exposed to a frightening level of risk that is now reported on the front pages of our newspapers at an alarmingly frequent rate. Every parent who considers allowing a child to play football, hockey, or any other contact sport needs to be aware of this information.

To younger adults, and especially for their children, there's no time like the present to listen up. Accumulating multiple injuries that begin in young age is a set-up for problems later in life. Simple injuries like muscle strains and even bone fractures will heal with time if properly treated. They can heal to be nearly as good as pre-injury. But repetitive injury will eventually take its toll, especially with injuries to joints, the spine, and, as we now know, the brain. Despite everything I've written here, I still hesitate to advise parents to stop their children from playing football, or any other contact sport. There are good aspects of all sports, other than boxing. Some children, both boys and girls, are drawn to sport, and it can be the primary focus of their scholastic achievement. It can help get you into college and for the truly gifted, provide a scholarship.

I would, however, recommend a one-concussion limit. Any child concussed in a youth contact sport should not return to that sport. Head injury can, of course, occur in any sport or exercise, contact or otherwise, but it's less likely in the non-contact ones. There is no reason to up the ante and needlessly subject the young brain to an unnecessary risk of re-injury. I doubt that the national psyche is ready at this point to heed that advice. It's equally unlikely that adults who are concussed in recreational sports will do so. Yet it is how I advise my patients and their parents. Some accept it, many don't. With time I suspect that attitudes will change, and the ratio of acceptance to non-acceptance will invert. Common sense backed by reliable research will ensure that.

I can imagine a time when scholastic and collegiate football will no longer exist. As the information about the dangers of mild head injury becomes more commonplace, increasing numbers of parents will keep their children away from full-contact sports. And as suing others for one's misfortune has become a favorite American pastime, the legal liability alone could put schools out of the football business. The immediate devastation of catastrophic head and spinal cord injuries uniformly finds its way into court, and the late effects of repetitive injuries, causing severe neurologic disability including early onset dementia, threatens to put the NFL into a legal tailspin. The number of plaintiffs in the current litigation brought by former NFL players has expanded dramatically since it was filed in 2012.

Given the penchant in government nowadays for protecting us from ourselves (witness New York mayor Michael Bloomberg's attempt to ban large-size soft drink containers), it seems likely that it's only a matter of time before there is legislative oversight of all contact sports. Libertarians will be howling. As I've said, however, the banning of boxing can't come too soon.

As I began my research into the sports and exercises with which I had little or no personal experience, I learned that, although occurrences are rare, even low-impact exercise and sports can cause serious injury, even death. And there is no correlation between how extreme a sport is and how severely one can be injured. More importantly, less devastating but still significantly life-altering injuries can occur with even moderate activities. It usually happens because we are unprepared, don't take precautions, don't train appropriately, and don't use adequate equipment. Add to that overzealous coaches and parents, poorly trained teachers, and trainers with little experience, and untoward events are inevitable.

The aging process takes an inevitable toll on the human body. Despite what Jack LaLanne and Charles Atlas told us, we become more injury-prone as we age. To my generation of baby boomers, I suggest looking in the mirror without the rose-colored glasses. We really don't look the same as we did all those years ago, except for my wife of course, who looks better than she did the day I met her in 1978. And if we don't look the same on the outside, the same goes for the inside, especially our spine, bones, joints, muscles, tendons, and ligaments. The more you push yourself, the more likely you are to hurt yourself, especially if you don't listen to your body. It's not brain surgery. It's actually quite simple. The good news for the boomers is that if you've made it to here in relatively good shape, it's likely due, at least in part, to the fact that you've taken good care of yourself and did indeed listen to your body. I do, and it's constantly telling me to relax and take it easy. And I do. Frequently.

And yes, don't eat too much. I do at times, despite my best intentions not to. Excess weight does so many bad things to the human body. Beyond the medical risks of obesity—diabetes, heart attack, and stroke are just a few of the many—is the added stress on our musculoskeletal system. Not a day goes by when I have office hours that I don't see someone who has chronic back pain and is significantly if not morbidly obese. In my head I hear myself screaming, "You need to stop over-eating, get off the couch, and lose weight!" I even tell them, gasp, that they should exercise a little. If I actually say only that, the patient storms out of my office, creates a stir in my waiting room, and writes a scathing letter to my hospital's chief-of-staff. In today's digital age it's also likely to get you trashed on an internet physician evaluation site. So much for the truth.

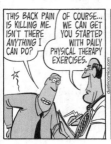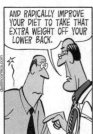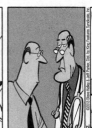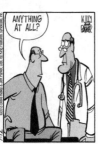

Instead of choosing to change their behavior to solve their problem, the patient wants a detailed anatomic explanation of what's at the root of their pain, what medications, therapy, or surgery will cure them, and how soon I can get it started. If I slip into the conversation that they "carry a few extra pounds" and recommend that the physical therapist working on their back can help them lose some weight, they are far more accepting. If I've learned anything in thirty-six years of seeing such patients, it's that diplomacy has a role in medicine too.

I also caution them to be wary of the hyperbole coming from the purveyors of vitamins, nutritional supplements, fad diets, no-effort exercise machines, and herbal remedies. In many cases, the claims of the advantages of these products are at best exaggeration and at worst cynical scams. If the government ever contemplates anything as controversial as banning youth contact sports, it should certainly consider tighter oversight of the unproven claims of the nutrition industry. The medical experts who have become national celebrities hawking these products should be ashamed of themselves. In academic circles they are considered opportunists and are not taken seriously.

My personal revelation came with my bicycle injury, the fractured wrist that happened without an accident. It's one thing to enjoy a sport with full recognition that there is risk that can produce injury. It's quite another to get blindsided by happenstance. It made me realize how little control we actually have over the possible consequences of our activities. One can take every precaution, train appropriately, buy the best equipment and still end up injured. Exercise will hurt you. It's only a matter of time.

So there it is. Stay active, don't eat too much, and above all, use common sense. All things in moderation, goes the classic piece of advice. It's good advice. It should be applied to how we exercise, how we participate in sports, how we eat and, most importantly, how we treat our bodies.

I hope my thoughts have advanced the cause of that common sense.

One of my favorite prayers gives thanks for our having been given life, for being kept in health, and for bringing us to joyous occasions.

May it always be so.

NOTES

INTRODUCTION

1. Gretchen Reynolds, "Can You Get Too Much Exercise," *New York Times* online, July 24, 2013.

2. Kasper Anderson, Bahman Farahmand, Anders Ahlbom, Claes Held, Sverker Ljunghall, Karl Michaelsson and Johan Sundstrom, "Risk of arrhythmias in 52,755 long-disance cross-country skiers: a cohort study," *European Heart Journal*, first published online: June 11, 2013 doi:10.1093/eurheartj/eht188.

3. Reynolds, *New York Times* on-line, July 24, 2013.

4. M. Wilson, R. O'Hanlon, S. Prasad, A. Deighan, P. Macmillan, D. Oxborough, R. Godfrey, G. Smith, A. Maceira, S. Sharma, K. George and G. Whyte, "Diverse patterns of myocardial fibrosis in lifelong, veteran endurance athletes," *Journal of Applied Physiology*, 2011 June; 110(6): 1622-6, doi: 10.1152/japplphysiol.01280.2010.

5. E. Gausch, B. Benito, X. Qi, P. Naud, Y. Shi, A. Mighiu, A. Tadevosyan, Y. Chen, MA. Gillis, YK. Iwasaki, D. Dobrev, L. Mont, S. Heximer, and S. Nattel, "Atrial fibrillation promoted by endurance exercise: demonstration and mechanistic exploration in an animal model," *Journal of the American College of Cardiology*, 2013 Jul 2;62(1):68-77, doi: 10.1016/j.jacc.2013.01.091.

6. H. Dor-Haim, O. Berenfeld, M. Horowitz, C. Lotan and M. Swissa, "Reduced ventricular arrhythmogeneity and increased electrical complexity in normal exercised rats," *PLoS ONE*, 8(6): e66658, doi: 10.1371/journal.pone.0066658.

7. U.S. Institute of Medicine, " To Err is Human: Building a Better Health Care System." *National Academy Press*, (Baltimore), 2008.

CHAPTER I: THE CULT OF EXERCISE

1. Thomas Vennun, *American Indian Lacrosse, The Little Brother of War*, Johns Hopkins University Press, (Baltimore), 2008.

2. Edward Hoffman, "The Moses Maimonides-Hoffman Wellness Survey," *Jerusalem Post Magazine*, March 5, 2010, http://www.jpost.com/Magazine/Personal-Notes/The Moses Maimonides-Hoffman-wellness-survey.

3. Wade Frazier, "Paul Bragg's Tarnished Legacy," May 2007, http://www.ahealedplanet.net/bragg.htm.

4. Richard Goldstein, "Jack LaLanne, Founder of Modern Fitness Movement, Dies at 96," *The New York Times*, January 23, 2011.

5. Ibid.

6. Jonathan Black, "Charles Atlas: Muscle Man," *Smithsonian Magazine*, August, 2009, Vol. 40, No. 5, 66.

7. Black, 66.

8. Black, 66.

9. Black, 67.

10. Black, 68.

11. Jack Holland, "How Much Money Americans Spend For Gym Memberships," coolefitness.com, November 27, 2012.

12. Ibid.

13. Yang, Jingzhen; Tibbetts, Abigail S.; Covassin, Tracey; Cheng, Gang; Nayar, Saloni; Heiden, Erin; "Epidemiology of overuse and acute injuries among competitive

collegiate athletes," *Journal of Athletic Training*, 2012 Mar-Apr; 47(2): 198-204. ISSN: 1062-6050 PMID: 22488286.

14. Albright JP; Powell JW; Martindale A; Black R; Crowley E; Schmidt P; Monroe J; Locy D; Aggler T; Davis WR; et al.; "Injury patterns in Big Ten Conference football," *American Journal of Sports Medicine*, 2004 Sep; 32 (6): 1394-404. ISSN: 0363-5465 PMID: 15310563.

15. Yang, Ibid.

16. Clarsen, Benjamin; Myklebust, Grethe; Bahr, Roald; "Development and validation of a new method for the registration of overuse injuries in sports injury epidemiology: the Oslo Sports Trauma Center (OSTRC) Overuse Injury Questionnaire," *British Journal of Sports Medicine*, 2013 May; 47 (8): 495-502. ISSN: 0306-3674 PMID: 23038786

17. Bahr R; "No injuries, but plenty of pain? On the methodology for recording overuse symptoms in sports," *British Journal of Sports Medicine*, 2009 Dec; 43 (13): 966-72. ISSN: 0306-3674 PMID: 19945978.

18. W.-C Tsai, F.-T Tang, C.-C Hsu, Y.-H Hsu, J.-H. S. Pang, and C.-C. Shiue, "Ibuprofen inhibition of tendon cell proliferation and upregulation of the cyclin kinase inhibitor p21CIP1," *Journal of Orthopaedic Research*, vol. 22, no. 3, 2006, 586-591.

19. L.C. Almekinders, A.J. Baynes, and L. W. Bracey, "An in vitro investigation into the effects of repetitive motion and nonsteroidal anti-inflammatory medication on human tendon fibroblasts," *American Journal of Sports Medicine*, vol. 23, no. 1, 1995, 119-123.

20. S.T. Ferry, L.E. Dahners, H.M. Afshari, and P.S. Weinhold, "The effect of common anti-inflammatory drugs on the healing rat patellar tendon," *American Journal of Sports Medicine*, vol 35, no. 8, 2007, 1326-1333.

CHAPTER 2: RECREATIONAL, FASHIONABLE EXERCISE

1. R Ferber, A Hreljac, and KD Kendall, "Suspected mechanisms in the cause of overuse running injuries: a clinical review," *Sports Health*, vol. 1, no. 3, May 2009, 242-6.

2. JF Decalzi, SJ Narvy, CT Vangsness Jr, Overview of cycling injuries: results of a cycling club survey. *Orthopedics*, 2013 Apr; 36 (4): 287-9. ISSN: 0147-7447 PMID: 23590771.

3. Ibid.

4. SL Castle, RV Burke, MP Arbogast, JS Upperman, "Bicycle helmet legislation and injury patterns in trauma patients under age 18," J Surg Res. 2012; 173(2):327-331.

5. V Tan, RM Seldes, A Daluiski, "In-line skating injuries.," *Sports Med*. 2001; 31(9):691-699.

6. KM Rosenkranz, RL Sheridan "Trauma to adult bicyclists: a growing problem in the urban environment," *Injury*, 2003; 34(11):825-829.

7. JM Conn, JL Annest, J Gilchrist, "Sports and recreation related injury episodes in the US population, 1997-99," *Inj Prev*, 2003; 9(2):117-123.

8. "101 Inventions that Changed the World," The History Channel, aired July 7, 2013.

9. Melissa Dribben, "Jumping into what you know is a downward trip," *The Philadelphia Inquirer*, July 7, 2013.

10. Stephen Miller, "Fred Epstein, 68, Leading Pediatric Neurosurgeon," *New York Sun*, July 12, 2006.

11. William J. Broad, "How Yoga Can Wreck Your Body," *The New York Times*, January 5, 2012.

12. Ibid.

13. Ibid.

14. W. Ritchie Russell, "Yoga and the Vertebral Arteries," *British Medical Journal*, vol. 1, no. 5801, March 11, 1972.

15. Arlene A. Schmid, et al., "Poststroke Balance Improves With Yoga," *Stroke*, July 26, 2012.

16. Babylonian Talmud Tractate Sanhedrin 37a

CHAPTER 3: COMPETITIVE, CONTACT EXERCISE

1. A.J. Liebling, *The Sweet Science* (New York: Farrar, Straus and Giroux, 2004); Bert Randolph Sugar, *One Hundred Years of Boxing: A Pictorial History of Modern Boxing, 1882–1982*, (New York: Smithmark Publishers 1982.)

2. George D. Lundberg, MD, "Boxing Should Be Banned in Civilized Countires," *The Journal of the American Medical Association*, January 14, 1983.

3. KM Guskiewicz, SW Marshall, J Bailes, M McCrea, RC Cantu, C Randolph, BD Jordan, "Association between recurrent concussion and late-life cognitive impairment in retired professional football players," *Neurosurgery*, vol. 57, no. 4, October 2005, 719-26.

4. KM Guskiewicz, SW Marshall, J Bailes, M McCrea, HP Harding, A. Matthews Jr., JR Mihalik, RC Cantu, "Recurrent concussion and risk of depression in retired professional football players," *Medicine & Science in Sports & Exercise*, vol. 39, no. 6, June 2007, 903-9.

5. "Dementia Pugilistica," *Boxrec Boxing Encyclopedia*, May 1, 2009, boxrec.com.

6. Nick Meyer, "How the Advent of the Forward Pass in College Football Saved Lives," *Yahoo! Voices*, September 12, 2007. http://voices.yahoo.com/how-advent-forward-pass-college-football-544858.html?cat=14.

7. "History," National Collegiate Athletic Association, accessed July 8, 2013, www.ncaa.org.

8. Mike Jensen and Robert Moran, "Autopsy: Penn star had brain disease," *The Philadelphia Inquirer*, September 14, 2010.

9. Jack Kelly, "Sports head injuries can ignite brain overreaction," *Pittsburgh Post-Gazette*, September 19, 2011

10. P. McCrory, W. Meeuwisse, J. Kutcher, B. Jordan and A. Gardner, "What is the evidence for chronic concussion-related changes in retired athletes: behavioural, pathological

and clinical outcomes?" *British Journal of Sports Medicine*, 2013; 47:327-330. doi:10.1136/bjsports-2013-092248.

11. Ibid.

12. N. Virji-Babul, M. Borich, N. Makan, T. Moore, K. Frew, C. Emery and L. Boyd, "Diffusion tensor imaging of sports-related concussion in adolescents," *Pediatric Neurology*, 2013; 48: 24-29. doi.org/10.1016/j.pediatrneurol.2012.09.005.

13. Ibid.

14. H.S.Martland,"PunchDrunk,"JAMA,1928;91(15):1103-1107. doi:10.1001/jama.1928.02700150029009

15. McCrory, et.al., Ibid.

16. Ibid.

17. KM Guskiewicz, SW Marshall, J Bailes, M McCrea, RC Cantu, C Randolph, BD Jordan, "Association between recurrent concussion and late-life cognitive impairment in retired professional football players," *Neurosurgery*, vol. 57, no. 4, October 2005, 719-26.

18. KM Guskiewicz, SW Marshall, J Bailes, M McCrea, HP Harding, A. Matthews Jr., JR Mihalik, RC Cantu, "Recurrent concussion and risk of depression in retired professional football players," *Medicine & Science in Sports & Exercise*, vol. 39, no. 6, June 2007, 903-9.

19. McCrory, et.al., Ibid.

20. Ann McKee, MD, and Robert Cantu, MD, "TDP-43 Proteinopathy and Motor Neuron Disease in Chronic Traumatic Encephalopathy," *Journal of Neuropathology and Experimental Neurology*, vol. 69, no. 9, September 2010, 918 – 929.

21. Ibid.

22. John P. Martin, "Hearing Tuesday in concussion lawsuit against NFL," *Philadelphia Inquirer*, April 7, 2013.

23. Anna Stolley Persky, "Playing It Safe: Are Concussions Ruining Sports?" *Washington Lawyer*, vol. 27, No.8, April 2013.

24. Ken Belson, "NFL agrees to settle concussion suit for $765 million," *The New York Times*, August 29, 2013.

25. Ken Belson, "Many ex-players may be ineligible for payment in N.F.L. concussion settlement," *The New York Times*, October 17, 2913.

26. Editorial, "Timely heads-up on NFL injuries," *The Philadelphia Inquirer*, January 19, 2014.

27. Ann McKee, MD, and Robert Cantu, MD, "TDP-43 Proteinopathy and Motor Neuron Disease in Chronic Traumatic Encephalopathy," *Journal of Neuropathology and Experimental Neurology*, vol. 69, no. 9, September 2010, 918 – 929.

28. MJ Winder, K Brett, and RJ Hurlbert, "Spinal cord concussion in a professional hockey player," *Journal of Neurosurgery. Spine*, vol. 14, no. 5, May 2011, 677–80, doi:10.3171/2011.1.SPINE10345.

29. Ibid.

30. D. Pang and J.E. Wilberger, "Spinal cord injury without radiographic abnormalities in children." *Journal of Neurosurgery*, vol. 57, 1982, 114–129, doi: 10.3171/jns.1982.57.1.0114.

CHAPTER 4: EXTREME EXERCISE

1. EH Gombrich, *A Little History of the World* (New Haven: Yale Univeristy Press, 2008), 39.

2. Ibid.

3. Peter McKenzie-Brown, "The Story of the Marathon," *Impact*, March 2010.

4. SC Matthews, DL Narotsky, et al., "Mortality among marathon runners in the United States, 2000-2009," *The American Journal of Sports Medicine*, vol. 40, no. 7, July 2012, 1495–500.

5. Ibid.

6. "The Dangers of Extreme Sports," rational worldview .com, August 5. 2013.

7. Ibid.
8. Ibid.
9. Ibid.
10. Ibid.
11. Ibid.
12. J. Upton, "CrossFit:Cult of Conditioning Program," *U.S. News and World Report*, July 31, 2012.
13. Ibid.
14. S. Cooperman, "Getting Fit, Even if it Kills You," *New York Times*, December 22, 2005.
15. Ibid.
16. J. V. Isaksen, "The Psychology of Extreme Sports: Addicts, Not Loonies," *Popular Social Science*, November 5, 2012.
17. Ibid.
18. Châu Belle, Williams Belle, Yann Hnautra, and Mark Daniels (Director) *Generation Yamakasi*, [TV documentary], France, 'France 2.'
19. "Why there are no Parkour competitions," Parkourpedia .com. Accessed July 10, 2013.
20. Ben Musholt, "Parkour Injuries: 2012 Survey Results," *Parkour Conditioning*, December 9, 2012. http://parkourconditioning.com/parkour-injuries-survey/.
21. Ibid.
22. Nate Berg, "Parkour Is Not A Crime (Except When It Is)," *The Atlantic Cities*, November 29, 2011. http://www.theatlanticcities.com/arts-and-lifestyle/2011/11/parkour-not-crime/598/ Nate Berg 11/29/11
23. "Lisa J. Huriash, "Parkour participants looking for a home in Margate," *Sun Sentinel*, November 28, 2011. http://articles.sun-sentinel.com/2011-11-28/news/fl-margate-extreme-sports-20111128_1_parkour-margate-mayor-pam-donovan-city-parks.
24. Associated Press, "At Nebraska's Stadium, Researchers Will Take Aim at Making Sports Safer." *The New York Times*, July 6, 2013.

25. Ibid.
26. Debate Club, "Should Football Be Fundamentally Changed to Make It Safer?" *U.S. News and World Report*, February 1, 2013.
27. Ibid.
28. D. Remick, "Going the Distance On and off the road with Barack Obama," *The New Yorker*, January 27, 2014.

CHAPTER 5: THE SPORTS-INDUSTRIAL COMPLEX

1. Dwight D. Eisenhower, "The Farewell Address," The Eisenhower Institute, Gettysburg College, January 17, 1961. Accessed July 10. http://www.eisenhowerinstitute.org/.
2. "The Business of College Sports," *Top Business Degrees*, http://www.top-business-degrees.net/college-sports/. Accessed July 11, 2013.
3. David Zirin, "What's My Name, Fool? Sports and Resistance in the United States," (Chicago: Haymarket Books, 2005), 17.
4. WR Hambrecht + Co. Sports Finance Group, "The U.S. Professional Sports Market & Franchise Value Report 2012," 2012, accessed July 15, 2013, http://www.wrhambrecht.com/pdf/SportsMarketReport_2012.pdf.
5. J. George, "What are the Eagles Worth?" *Philadelphia Business Journal*, August 14, 2013
6. D. Sirota, "The sports-industrial complex is bleeding America dry," Salon.com, February 13, 2013
7. N. Mills, "The sports-industrial complex," The Guardian .com, December 9 2007.
8. Ibid.
9. N. McNerney, "Dealing with the Athletic Industrial Complex," Reducehomeworkstress.com, December 26, 2011.
10. Ibid.
11. Ibid.
12. Mark Scolforo, "Graham Spanier Suing Louis Freeh For Slander Over Report On Sandusky Cover Up," *Huffington Post*, July 11, 2013.

CHAPTER 6: WHAT DO I DO?

1. "50 Germiest Places in the World," *Forensic Science Technician: Online Schools Guide*, http://www.forensicsciencetechnician.org/50-germiest-places-in-the-world/.   Accessed July 10, 2013.

CREDITS AND PERMISSIONS

Scaphoid bone and illustration of screw in scaphoid bone, page 12, courtesy of American Society for Surgery of the Hand.

Caution sticker from ladder, page 23, courtesy of the author.

Anatomy of the Knee, page 42, Bruce Blaus, Wikicommons.

Structure of skeletal muscle fiber, page 48, copyright © Alila Medical Media.

Sliding Filament Model of Muscle Contraction, page 51, copyright © OpenStax College, Anatomy & Physiology, http://cnx.org/content/col11496/1.6/.

Peroneal Nerve at the Knee, page 92, Image reprinted with permission from Medscape Reference http://emedicine.medscape.com, 2014, available at: http://emedicine.medscape.com/article/1234607-overview.

Cerebral vasculature, page 93, originally appeared in Renan Uflackerm, *Atlas of Vascular Anatomy*, (Wolters Kluwer Health, 2006), reprinted with permission.

Nerve Cell, page 105, Nicolas Rougier, Wikicommons.

Neuronal Interconnections, page 107, image courtesy of

the National Institute on Aging/National Institutes of Health.

Scans of Diffuse Axonal Injury (DAI), page 112, copyright © Alila Medical Media.

MRI of DAI, page 112, Hellerhoff, Wikicommons.

CSF Circulation, page 114, copyright © OpenStax College, Anatomy & Physiology, http://cnx.org/content/col11496/1.6/.

CTE Injury, page 125, reprinted from American Academy of Physical Medicine and Rehabilitation, Vol 3, Robert A. Stern, PhD et al., Long-term Consequences of Repetitive Brain Trauma: Chronic Traumatic Encephalopathy, S462, 2011, with permission from Elsevier.

Owen Thomas, page 126, image courtesy of Penn Athletics.

Juinor Seau, page 126, AP Photo/Elaine Thompson.

Spinal Injury Scale, page 148, copyright © Alila Medical Media.

Dustin comic, page 223, DUSTIN © 2013 Steve Kelley & Jeff Parker, Dist. By King Features Syndicate, Inc.